# Hygge

## Discovering the Danish Art of Happiness

*(Introduce Unending Happiness to Your Home With Art of Hygge)*

**Gordon Wilkinson**

Published By **Jordan Levy**

# Gordon Wilkinson

*Hygge: Discovering the Danish Art of Happiness
(Introduce Unending Happiness to Your Home
With Art of Hygge)*

**ISBN 978-1-998927-90-6**

Legal & Disclaimer

# Table Of Contents

# Chapter 1: Creating The Hygge Mood At Home

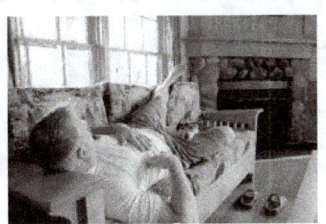

Using Natural Light In Your Space Effectively

We require herbal mild to be glad and healthful. It heightens our interest and complements our mood, productiveness, and mind-set. It substantially influences our body as it's how we produce weight-reduction plan D, that is critical for a robust immune device and bone density.

There are many techniques.

•To significantly growth the amount of natural moderate inside the residence, try replacing heavy voile or lace curtains with sheer panel coverings.

•Repaint the walls in mild grey, white, or cream to growth the texture of spaciousness.

•Place mirrors and smooth-surfaced furniture in strategic places to mirror slight and go back it into the room.

Try some of the ones tips, and you can see how a extraordinary, airy surroundings fosters tranquility.

Get Comfy And Cozy With Soft Furnishings

Nothing is extra romantic than curling up on a sofa covered in pillows and a warmth blanket or cover while it is cold out of doors.

You can get lost in a e-book, a film, or a nap at the identical time as cocooned in a layer of softness. Cover your sofa with merino wool, faux fur, cashmere cushions, throws, and blankets. These lovely textures are perfect for nesting into and right away upload warmth and richness to any area. Put to your coziest jammies and 2 wool socks to boom the hygge element.

# Introduce Some Nature Into Your Home

Our bodies and minds advantage from nature's calming results, which additionally help to create a welcoming environment. There are severa strategies to introduce individual interior. The brilliant locations to start are indoor flora and freshly cut plants. They add brightness and exquisite smells to any area.

Pick some vegetation from your outside and located them in jam jars for a country look. You can also gather appealing stones, shells, and driftwood. You can also construct table decorations out of bark, leaves, berries, and pine cones which you accumulated on a walk within the nation-state or alongside the coast. Pebbles, domestic made ceramics, natural timber floors, and furnishings all upload relaxed, herbal textures to a area.

Using herbal materials ought to make it clean to make your private home appearance lovable and connected to the environment outdoors.

# Breath In The Fresh Air

Numerous houseplants are exceptional air purifiers for homes. They purify your property's air by manner of getting rid of volatile pollutants and contaminants. The following vegetation are the first-class-purchased air-filtering vegetation.

It could be a remarkable idea to preserve this form of vegetation inside a hundred square ft of your own home or condominium:

- Aloe vera.

- Palm bamboo (Dypsis lutescens)

- Boston fern (Nephrolepis exaltata)

- Banana palm (Musa basjoo)

- Barberton daisy (Gerbera jamesonii)

- Broadleaf woman palm (Rhapis excelsa)

- Mandarin evergreen (Aglaonema)

- English ivy (Hedera helix)

- Flamingo lily

- Elephant ear philodendron (Philodendron domesticum)

- Devil's ivy (Epipremnum aureum) (Anthurium andraeanum)

- Flowershop daisy (Chrysanthemum morifolium)

- Lily grass (Liriope muscari)

- Kimberly queen fern (Nephrolepis obliterate)

- Heart-leaf philodendron (Philodendron cordatum);

- Moth orchids (Phalaenopsis)

- Peace lily; (Spathiphyllum)

Enjoying Open Fires

One of life's great pleasures is unwinding inside the the the front of a fire. Whether in the front of an open fireplace or a contemporary-day-day wood burner, a log fireside's crackles and flickering flames produce a heat, inviting ambiance. The soothing scent of wood smoke induces emotions of calmness and contentment, crucial connection, and a enjoy of network.

The fireplace serves as the focal point and the middle of the house, wherein recollections are informed, and occasions are celebrated. Invite loved ones and buddies to spend time together spherical the fireside gambling easy pleasures like roasting marshmallows or gambling video video games, or surely loosen up and take in the splendor of the dancing flames.

Storing And Stacking Firewood

If you have a wood-burning stove or open fireside, you're in all likelihood aware about how essential it's miles to have sufficient logs available to get you thru the bloodless iciness months. One of the copious definitions of hygge is taking detail in a warmth fireplace on the equal time as sitting down. But did you apprehend that successfully stacked firewood is essential for a fire to burn efficiently?

How to correctly hasten timber drying

To hasten drying, first purchase logs that have been cut up into short lengths, ideally 10 inches (25 cm) long. Then preserve your logs in a log preserve that has well air glide. Many people make the error of piling the logs at the ground and protecting them with a tarp, but doing so promotes the growth of mildew and deterioration. One of the maximum essential factors in retaining your firewood dry is air flow into. Therefore, shopping a log keep pays off because it permits the timber to be stored above the floor.

It want to have a roof over the top and be ethereal on the rims. Place the log garage at the house's blanketed aspect. Your wooden must be stacked in rows with regions amongst them to promote airflow. Leave about 4 inches (10 cm) maximum of the logs and the floor if stacking towards a wall or fence. The most critical component of properly-stacked timber is that it will probable be satisfactory and dry even as you want it.

Dry wooden burns more successfully and produces lots less smoke. Note: Dry firewood is never in short deliver in a heat, comfortable, hyggelig home!

Setting Up The Table

Setting a lovely table does no longer surely need to be for unique activities; you may do it daily to make every meal memorable. It does not must be pricey; paper or linen napkins and a simple white tablecloth, in addition to currently-picked vegetation in a jam jar, a twig of fall leaves, or a tough and rapid of beach treasures organized inside the middle of the desk, produce a smooth but appealing final outcomes.

Glass and candles straight away provide shine and environment. When web hosting a meeting, do not worry about making the entirety best; a smooth spread of cheeses, olives, bread, and wine, or perhaps only some baked buns, will display off the affection and care you located into your meal.

## Lighting Up The Candles

Danish people burn extra candles everyday with individual than some exclusive Europeans for a excellent reason: sharing hyggelig moments is essential at the same time as enduring the awful Scandinavian winters and leaden skies, and lighting candles is one of the best strategies to create a warm temperature and alluring atmosphere.

Place lanterns, candles, and tea lighting fixtures during your own home—next on your computer, spherical the hearth, and on the eating room desk—the greater glowing lights, the higher. Place your candles cautiously because some detail which could begin a fire interior your own home can be dangerous. This list of critical dos and don'ts will make sure which you stay strong:

Do:

•You need to keep candles out of the direction of curtains, fabric, and distinctive overhanging gadgets.

•To ensure that candles are held erect and may not tip over, region them within the proper holders.

•You want to commonly area candles on a heatproof ground. You want to use tea lighting with more warning because of the truth that they might get heat enough to melt plastic.

•You must constantly manipulate candles cautiously thinking about that they grow to be liquid even as lit. Place them on a steel or glass plate.

•Make certain that youngsters and pets cannot get your candles.

Don't Do:

•If you perhaps go away the room, do not leave the candles burning.

•Because clothing and hair can quick capture hearth, never lean over a candle.

•It may additionally help if you did not place a candle under a shelf because of the reality it could without problems burn the floor's underside.

•Don't blow out a candle while placing it out because of the fact doing so can reason heat wax and sparks to fly. To placed it out, use a spoon or a snuffer.

•Never allow a teenager go to sleep with a burning candle or oil burner of their bed room.

•Avoid shifting a burning candle— continuously snuff out the flame first.

Different Waxes

Paraffin wax is used to make the bulk of candles. A spinoff of crude oil, paraffin wax is frequently blended with chemical substances to growth burn pace. Many people fear that burning the ones candles can also generate toxic black soot and unique air pollutants. Alternative waxes burn purifier and produce a wonderful deal much less smoke and soot.

Although beeswax charges greater than paraffin wax, it's far a natural wax made via honeybees. Another opportunity is soybean-derived soy wax. It may be made completely of soybean oil, it virtually is much less costly than beeswax, or you can combination it with special vegetable oils or waxes.

Essential Oils

Purchase candles with important oil infusions. Essential oils can impact our thoughts, feelings, and moods, beautify our well-being, and infuse the gap with lovable scents. Different oils have one-of-a-kind results on us. Some important oils are a laugh, like lavender and bergamot, at the equal time as others are energizing, like lemon and rose.

If you're likely handling any of the under unfavourable health troubles, attempt a number of the subsequent:

•Insomnia: lavender, chamomile, jasmine, rose, and sandalwood

•Stress: lavender, bergamot, vetiver, pine, and ylang-ylang

•Anxiety: Roman chamomile, rose, clary sage, lemon, and sandalwood

•Depression: Chamomile, jasmine, peppermint, and chamomile

•Sage, peppermint, and cinnamon can assist with memory and attention problems.

•Clove, jasmine, tea tree, rosemary, sage, and citrus are low-energy flowers.

Clothing: Casual Is Key

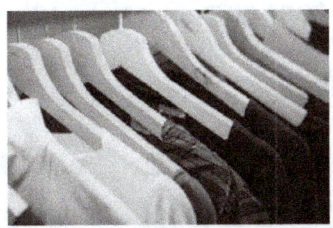

On Copenhagen's streets, you may now not see many three-piece suits, and if you're a member of the pinstriped commercial agency set, you will probable think the Danish dressing technique is downright messy. One can say that being casual and elegant on the

identical time is a Danish art work which you may in all likelihood discover ways to draw close through time.

Many human beings, which embody me, opt for the mixture of a T-shirt or sweater on the internal and a jacket on the outside for a informal but contemporary fashion. For coziness and the professor style, I love people with leather patches at the elbows.

My pals tease that within the event that they need to find me once I'm status with my again to them in a crowded pub, they handiest want to look at out for the patches, so I may also have a mild tendency to misuse the patches.

How To Dress Like A Dane

Danish fashion is streamlined, lovable, minimalistic, however no longer overly fussy. It actions a stability among minimalist, practical design, and hygge in lots of tactics.

Scarves

A headscarf is important. Both males and females are mission to this. Despite being especially used within the wintry climate, human beings with scarf withdrawal signs were seen the usage of scarves in the center of summer. The maxim is simple: the larger, the better. So cover your self in fashion with a densely wrapped headscarf, but be sure to stop quick of inflicting any neck damage.

Black

You may additionally assume that you have simply entered the set of a ninja movie as you go out the airport in Copenhagen. In Denmark, black is the dominant color. You need to head for a swish, monochromatic look that is probably suitable for Karl Lagerfeld's funeral. You can pick out from a wider variety of shades in the summer season, even a few difficulty outrageously ambitious like grey.

Top cumbersome

You can strike a stability amongst hygge and style with the useful resource of sporting hand-knitted wool sweaters, jumpers, cardigans, and pullovers on top, at the side of black leggings for girls and thin denims for men. Never put on sloppy sweaters; they may be cumbersome. Also, take into account the headband.

Layers

Layering is the call of the sport to enduring 4 seasons in within the destiny. Always have an additional cardigan with you. When you're freezing, hygge is impossible.

Woolen socks

As hygge insurance, arm your self with a beautiful pair of wool socks.

Casual hair

The Danish haircut is so casual that it nearly appears lazy. Get up and depart. For girls, a bun is an option; the better, the better.

Hygge Tip: How To Buy

Connect purchases to interesting stories. I had saved up cash for a state-of-the-art favorite chair, however I failed to buy it till after my first e-book changed into released. In this sense, the chair serves as a reminder of a outstanding victory I had.

You can use the identical not unusual sense for that particular sweater or those cute wool socks. When you located them on, you want to be reminded of that surely hyggelig 2nd, so save for them.

Togetherness

Creating cultures and life that manual the development of social interactions is vital. Naturally, focused on a healthy artwork-lifestyles balance is one solution. And on the subject of this, many humans are green with envy of Denmark. There is a lot of carefree contemplation whilst hygge is present.

Nobody monopolizes the speak or seizes the highlight for protracted periods of time.

Because everybody participates in the duties that make up the hyggelig night time, equality, a excellent this is firmly ingrained in Danish society, is a essential aspect of hygge. Instead of leaving the host on my own in the kitchen, it's miles more hyggelig if every body take part in the meal education.

Time spent with others cultivates a nice, laid-back, amiable, down-to-earth, near, relaxed, and welcoming surroundings. It resembles a excellent include in lots of respects, but with out bodily contact. You can be who you're and be in reality comfy in this condition. Therefore, extending your comfort location to encompass extraordinary humans is a part of the artwork of hygge.

Oxytocin: What's love had been given to do with it?

But at the same time as can we revel in having oxytocin circulating thru our our bodies? Hugs are often believed to make us happier, and this is actual—oxytocin begins offevolved to go together with the flow in near settings, which fosters human connection. As a cease end result, it's also called "the hormone of love" or "the hormone of cuddling."

Given that hygge is an intimate interest regularly associated with coziness and a few companionship, it stands to purpose that oxytocin might be released in those situations. Pet cuddles have the same effect as human cuddles in making us enjoy cherished, warmth, and safe—three of hygge's number one additives.

Since it fosters collaboration, take delivery of as actual with, and love among people, oxytocin—moreover referred to as "social glue"—is launched at the same time as we're bodily near some other person's body. Perhaps this explains why Danes have this kind of excessive diploma of keep in mind in fashionable strangers; they exercise hygge regularly due to the fact hyggelige sports cause the discharge of oxytocin, which reduces antagonism and fosters social connection.

This hormone is also released with the useful resource of heat and fullness. Candles, fires, warmness blankets, and delectable meals pass hand in hand with hygge. Hygge is, in a experience, all approximately oxytocin. Could it's that easy? Maybe it's now not a surprise that some aspect hygge-related makes us sense content material, comfortable, and steady.

The dark issue of hygge

There are clearly advantages to spending time along facet your near friends in a close to-knit social community in that you all have an extended facts collectively and are properly acquainted. However, in current years I actually have additionally come to understand that there may be a extreme drawback to any such social landscape: it isn't receptive to rookies.

I've heard the equal difficulty from each expat I've met who is settled in Denmark. The social circles there are almost not possible to enter. Or, at least, it necessitates years and years of diligence and perseverance. Admittedly, Danes struggle to consist of latest humans of their social networks.

This is in element because of the idea of hygge; if there were too many sudden faces at an event, it would be deemed an awful lot a whole lot less hyggeligt. It takes numerous artwork and loneliness along the way to sign up for a social corporation. The proper information is that, in my buddy Jon's phrases, "Once you are in, you are in," You can be assured that whilst you succeed, you will have made pals for life.

Hygge-socializing for introverts

It is properly identified that introverts get their electricity from internal, whilst extroverts get theirs from stimuli outside themselves. Extroverts are the people you want to hang out with in case you want to have a exceptional time; introverts are frequently perceived as loners. However, social gatherings aren't for everybody and might depart an introvert overstimulated and weary.

Social introverts do exist but the misconception that introversion is synonymous with shyness. (Just as calm extroverts do) This may also sound a chunk clichéd, but introverts often pick to devote their "social time" to loved ones whom they recognize thoroughly, to have excellent conversations, or to sit down down and examine a ebook with a few element heat to drink. This takes region to have a totally excessive hygge element—big, proper?

Introverts are social however in a extremely good way. There is not any unmarried manner of being social, but it'd feel like there are proper and incorrect techniques. Just because of the fact too many outdoor stimuli drain introverts does now not advocate they do not need to hang around with other people. With hygge, introverts may also additionally have a lovable, cushty middle of the night with a few buddies with out carrying out an entire lot of hobby or speaking to a huge group of people.

Hygge, it's an factor among mingling and fun, may be an opportunity for introverts who favor to live domestic as opposed to go to a huge birthday party with hundreds of strangers. It merges those worlds, that is exceptional for introverts and extroverts as it creates a middle ground.

Therefore, to all of you introverts available, please do not experience ashamed or fed up for having a preference for hygge-related objects. And to all the extroverts:

•Turn on some tender song.

•Light a few candles.

•For the middle of the night, encompass your inner introvert.

Hygge Tip: How to make recollections

We all agree that growing memories is the most sensitive a part of having them. Create a brand-new custom along with your circle of relatives or buddies. Two examples are the summer season solstice celebration by means of the use of way of the water or playing board video games at the primary Friday of every month. In reality, it can be any worthwhile activity that, over time, brings the organisation closer together.

## Chapter 2: Decorating Your Home

Hygge is ready developing a experience of

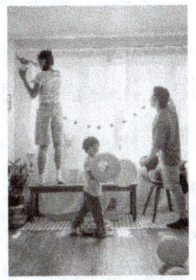

contentment and happiness; you do now not need to lay our a fortune to advantage this in your property. Decorate your home with matters that make you satisfied, like sparkling plant life. On u.S. Treks, you ought to build up plant life and pine cones. Add items as well. They carry up remarkable recollections, like paper snowflakes and seasonal bunting.

These small information make a house sense welcoming. When your internet site on line website online site visitors are happy, you may apprehend you've finished it effectively.

This is to say that they input through the door with a grin!

## Refreshing Flowers

Fresh vegetation are the excellent thing for the coronary heart and soul. Pick aromas that make you smile, like candy hyacinths or fragrant lilies, and beautify your home with blossoms that make you absolutely happy, which encompass bold tulips, romantic roses, and colourful daffodils. Hygge is about loving your self, so exit and deal with yourself to a bouquet of your preferred flowers as opposed to looking ahead to someone to shop for them for you.

Take easy peonies, lavender, and candy peas out of your window subject or garden. You can use jugs, jam jars, glass bottles, Mason jars, or even mugs in case you do not have enough vases. The flora ought to be located wherein you can see them every day, whether or not or no longer or not in a bouquet or genuinely one appealing stem.

## Creating A Natural Display

Do your wallet commonly include extremely good stones, twigs, and plant material at the same time as you get domestic from a stroll? Finding it hard to determine what to do with they all? If you make any discoveries, create a nature display at the same time as you get home. Have fun amassing your devices and contemplating ingenious methods to show off them.

You can also even put together a show using seashore driftwood and shells or fill glass jars with uncommon rocks and pebbles amassed from the seashore. When arranged in big vases or bowls, Berry branches and pine cones make a statement. These branches are big enough to be used as placing mobiles from the ceiling. Limit your show to greater than a touch desk within the corner.

Try arranging your treasures in a field or tray, or display them prominently on a mantelpiece or shelf. This is a lovely way to reconnect with nature's wonders, and the high-quality component is that the entire circle of relatives can participate. Happy collecting!

Things to accumulate

•Moss, pine cones, hazelnuts, twigs, fallen tree bark, chestnuts, sycamore helicopters, and acorns can be observed within the geographical area and the woods.

•Sunflower seed pods, dried sunflower seeds, dandelion clocks, stones, leaves, plant life, squash, and gourds are all decided in gardens.

•Shells (with out organisms interior), dried seaweed, seagull feathers, mermaid purses, and shark tooth can all be observed on the beach.

Paper Snowflakes

By developing the ones paper snowflakes, you could provide your desires for a snowy day. They're smooth to make and make your home appear to be a wintry weather wonderland. You can preserve them from the ceiling, string them collectively to create a garland, or affix them to windows to create a custom designed snow scene.

Making paper snowflakes will right away take you again in your childhood Christmases when they have been entire of appeal and wonder.

What you may want

•White square paper (mild-weight craft paper works terrific)

•Scalpel or razor-sharp scissors

Instructions

1.  Take one rectangular of paper. To create a triangle, fold the paper in half of of of diagonally.

2.  The triangle want to be folded two times, with the 2 sharp edges aligned. Proceed to fold the triangle into thirds (make certain the rims in shape up).

3.   Cutting directly at some stage inside the triangle's shortest element removes the triangle's two backside factors.

four.   Trim away shapes from the folded paper's edges. You should carefully open the paper to show your introduction.

Carving pumpkins

The surrender of October alerts one factor: it is time to get dressed in frightening clothing and carve pumpkins into lanterns! An fun social interest for own family and friends is pumpkin carving. The high-quality factor? A lit candle within the pumpkin will offer a lovely, comforting glow which will scare away witches and werewolves.

Instructions on a manner to carve a pumpkin

Use a pointy knife to reduce off the pumpkin's stem at the pinnacle considering it is extra tough than you may think.

Remove the flesh and seeds with a spoon; children experience this messy step. Save the seeds for destiny planting.

Use a felt-tip pen to attract or comedian strip a face or considered one of a kind layout onto the pumpkin. You ought to use a sharp knife to reduce out the patterns.

Insert a few natural or synthetic tea lights into the pumpkin. Place the stem returned on like a lid after lighting fixtures them.

Place your carved pumpkin out of doors at the doormat, a windowsill, or a gatepost to enchant guests and onlookers and brighten a dismal, bloodless nighttime.

Bunting In The Winter

Homemade bunting is a short and exciting manner to characteristic a festive surroundings to any indoor place. It offers a room a lovely border and a touch of captivating rusticity. It's easy to make, and you could use scraps of paper, portions of cloth, antique clothing, or maybe plastic and paper luggage to bring together your bunting. Have a calming craft day at domestic and allow your creativity run wild.

What you can need

•Cardboard (Thin)

•Attractive textiles and materials

•Glue or thread and needle

•String, twine, or ribbon

•To grasp the bunting, use drawing pins (non-obligatory)

•Scissors

Instructions

1.  Create a cardboard triangle template.

2.  Cut numerous triangles using the template from the cloth of your choice (wintry weather)—Tartan (as an example)

3.   Designs like snowflakes, icicles, and pine wood, further to warm colorings, work nicely.

4.   Attach the triangles to a bit of ribbon, thread, or natural wire the usage of glue or sewing.

five.   Deciding in which to hang your bunting is the maximum difficult step in the system! It complements the format of bedrooms and offers kitchens and dwelling regions a completely precise touch. As extended because it isn't always too close to the fireplace, you could hold it on walls, fasten it to shelves, or use it as a garland for a mantelpiece.

6.   Once your bunting is up, supply some pals to test it out (that is the precise pretext for an evening of board games, beverages, and snacks!).

Your Hygge Headquarters

Because our homes feature the center of hygge, the Danes are obsessed with indoors layout. In Denmark, social life revolves across the house. The social life of diverse global locations typically takes place in bars, ingesting places, and cafés, however the Danes choose hjemme hygge (home hygge), amongst different matters, due to the fact they don't like paying the excessive expenses in ingesting places.

According to a have a take a look at, seven out of ten Danes feel the most at home 'at domestic'. The Kähler Vase Scandal, additionally referred to as Vasegate, is arguably the clearest instance of the Danish hassle with layout. The Kähler vase modified right into a constrained model anniversary item that went on sale on August 25, 2014.

On that precise day, more than 16,000 Danes tried to shop for it online, maximum in useless for the motive that vase right away bought out. Long lineups of customers authentic outside the shops stocking the vase after the internet site failed. The limited deliver brought approximately a public outcry in competition to the agency that made the vase.

Hygge wishlist

- Cushions and blankets

- Vintage

- Think Tactile

- Ceramics

- Books

- Nature

- Things comprised of wood

- Candles

- A Fireplace

- A Hyggerkrog

Blankets and cushions


Any hygge home wants to embody blankets and pillows, particularly within the route of the chilly winter months. It's considerably hyggeligt to cuddle up with a blanket, and on occasion human beings do it even if they're now not cold because of the reality it's miles cozier. Fabrics like wool or fleece, which might be warmer, or cotton, which feels lighter, may be used to make blankets.

Cushions of all sizes are desired for hygge. What is probably greater comforting than analyzing your preferred e-book even as resting your head on a comfortable pillow? You are loose to move Freudian at the Danes at this point and observe that hygge appears to be targeted on consolation meals and comfortable blankets.

Vintage

Antique or retro stores are super locations to find out antique objects. It may be difficult to spot diamonds amid a sea of coal. A genuinely hyggeligt lamp, desk, or chair has visible better days. In a antique save, you can discover the whole thing they want to offer a beautiful domestic, and the gadgets internal are made all of the more interesting and cozier thru their history.

Many of these items play on testimonies and nostalgia. Objects have emotional clearly nicely worth and statistics similarly to their physical characteristics.

Think tactile

Your hyggelig indoors isn't always pretty a lot how matters appear, as you can have already observed out, but moreover how they experience. It feels very one-of-a-kind to the touch whatever made from metal, glass, or plastic than it does to run your arms throughout a hardwood table, over a heat ceramic cup, or via the hairs of a reindeer's pores and pores and skin. Add plenty of textures to your own home and do not forget how topics sense to the touch.

Ceramics

They are all attractive, whether or not or not a suitable teapot, a vase on the dining room desk, or your pass-to mug. Two of the maximum famous Danish ceramic producers are Kähler, which has a data courting returned more than one hundred seventy five years.

It made a huge influence on the Universal Exposition in Paris in 1889—the only 12 months the Eiffel Tower become inaugurated—and Royal Copenhagen, mounted in 1775 underneath the patronage of Queen Juliane Marie. This has in recent times expert a resurgence in recognition way to the Blue Fluted Mega range.

Books


Who could now not revel in a shelf stacked immoderate with weighty books? One of the pillars of the hygge philosophy is unwinding with an terrific e-book. No count the style, romance, technological information fiction, cooking manuals, or maybe horror reminiscences are welcome on the cabinets.

Every ebook is comfortable, but super works through writers like Jane Austen, Charlotte Bronte, Leo Tolstoy, and Charles Dickens have a totally particular place inside the library. When they may be vintage enough, your youngsters might also revel in reading aloud to them while they may be curled up subsequent to you within the hyggekrog.

Nature

Wood is inadequate. The complete forest must be delivered interior for the Danes. Any little little bit of nature you encounter is going to be taken into consideration hygge. Animal skins, twigs, leaves, nuts, and plant life. Essentially, you want to expect: How could a Viking squirrel decorate a residing room?

To upload even extra hygge, cowl those window sills, benches, and chairs in sheepskin. Sheep and reindeer may be alternated, at the equal time as cowhide is reserved for the ground. Copenhagen has been burned to the floor multiple instances, which is not surprising given the Danes' penchant for candles, wood, and different flammable substances.

Things made from timber

There is a few difficulty approximately timber devices that may be a hankering for our origins. The easy enjoy of a wooden bureau, the quiet creak of a hardwood floor as you stumble throughout it to take a seat within the wooden chair via the window, the smell of burning wooden from a hearth, or maybe a suit.

After years of plastic toys, wooden kid's toys are definitely in call for. An awesome instance of this is the timber monkey by using way of Kay Bojesen. Wood brings us inside the path of nature given that it's far simple and organic, just like the hygge aesthetic.

Candles

No candles, no hygge, it is just as smooth as that. Why may additionally moreover you be thinking? This is because of the fact hygge is targeted spherical creating a warmness and snug surroundings that may be without problems attained through having some candlelights lit.

Fireplace

I had a fortunate adolescence. The house I befell to grow up in had a wood-burning variety and an open hearth. My favored formative years obligation modified into to stack the wooden and begin the fireplace. I do not assume I'm the simplest one, even though. There are 28 million homes in the u . S .. What motivates the Danish manner of lifestyles's preoccupation with burning wood, then?

I'm effective   the solution to this one, however it couldn't only be approximately hygge, ought to it?. It is less expensive to say that a fire can be the ultimate hygge headquarters. It's a place wherein we spend time with our loved ones to deepen our experience of network and in which we sit down with the aid of way of ourselves to rest while experiencing the last sentiments of comfort and warmth.

A Hyggekrog

The one difficulty each house should have is a hyggekrog, that is Danish for "a nook." It's the room area in that you pick to curl up with a e-book, a cup of tea, and a blanket. Mine is with the beneficial aid of the window inside the kitchen. There are numerous pillows, a blanket, and a cowl from a reindeer there, and I additionally use it as a workspace at night.

Indeed, a huge thing of those pages became written there. Danes adore their relaxed surroundings. Hyggekrog is famous in Copenhagen and across the kingdom, and everybody wishes one. As you walk through the metropolis, you'll see that many structures feature bay home windows.

The inhabitants may want to have a snug spot to sit down and unwind after a hard day in those indoors areas, which might be nearly in truth equipped with pillows and blankets. However, although it's a long way hyggeligt, you do no longer ought to have your hyggekrog there. It may be a phase of a room.

You might also moreover create your hyggekrog in your own home, in which you can unwind with a notable ebook and some problem to drink, thru together with cushions or splendid snug gadgets to take a seat down on, mild lighting fixtures, and possibly a blanket. In Denmark, developing hyggeligt is a huge issue. To sell homes, some actual belongings shops even utilize hyggekrog.

# Chapter 3: Items That You Can Craft For Instant Hygge

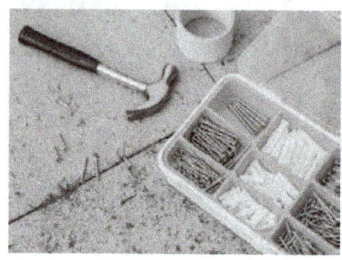

Making some thing from scratch along with your arms is among life's most pleasant joys. Whether you are making a fluffy pair of slippers or a adorable wooly cap with a pom-pom. Anything accomplished through the use of way of hand exudes man or woman and originality. The next pages show off the manner to create comfortable accessories and considerate gadgets that make you experience comfortable and content material cloth cloth.

Fairy-mild lanterns

Make some fairy-mild lanterns to carry a few glimmer into your life. Using fairy lights is a incredible way to set a wonderful mood. They offer off a dreamy, whimsical glow and supply every area a touch of attraction. Making those lanterns only takes a few minutes, providing a lovely backdrop for a party or a pleasant night time time in.

What you'll need

•1 to three huge Mason jars

•1-three strings of LED fairy lighting fixtures powered thru manner of batteries

•One piece large sufficient to cowl the battery percentage of sticky burlap tape

Instructions

1. Use a scrap of burlap to cover the battery % in a unmarried string of fairy lighting fixtures. Make sure the on/off button goes through up so that you can speedy obtain in and turn the lighting fixtures off earlier than

carefully placing the battery % into the bottom of a mason jar.

2. Distribute the fairy lights in some unspecified time in the future of the jar to cowl the interior. (If you are the usage of a specially massive jar, you'll likely need to apply more than one strings of fairy lighting.)

three. Tape the mild string's pinnacle to the inner of the lid and then screw the jar's cap returned on.

four. You can choose to function a pink ribbon to the jar or leave it easy for a extra natural appearance.

5. Set the mason jar(s) on a tray or mantelpiece and decorate the bottom with pine cones, decorations, and confetti stars.

6. Take a step decrease back and respect your introduction.

Note: An opportunity is to purchase a string of fairy lights with a battery p.C. That fits snugly sufficient to be taped to the jar lid. To hide the battery percentage, affix a thick piece of cloth or ribbon to the jar's neck.

Mug relaxed

Make your selected mug a savvy little jacket for wintry climate—now not only will it appearance very fetching, but it'll furthermore keep your heat chocolate steaming a hint bit longer. It's furthermore a genius way to upcycle a wooly sock!

What you may need

•Ruler

•Mug

•Wooly socks

•Needle and thread

•Scissors

•Fabric glue (Optional)

•Button felt shapes, mini-pom-poms, and sequins are optionally available gildings

47

Instructions

1.  Select your chosen cup and gauge its top.

2.   Keep the top part of the sock and decrease it off on the ankle.

three.   You want to turn the pinnacle of the sock inner out and use the thread to hem the seams firmly.

4.   Cut a slit for the cup cope with after turning the sock indoors out.

five.   To save you the edges from fraying, both overstitch them or take a look at fabric glue. If the use of glue, use remarkable a tiny amount so it will dry smooth, and allow it dry for the amount of time endorsed on the bottle. Fit your snug over the cup after that.

6.   By including progressive prospers the use of buttons, felt, or some thing else your creativity allows, you may supply your cup cushty a chunk greater hygge. Why save you there, then? To save you your flask from

feeling omitted, create a snug for it in addition.

Pom-Pom for a Beanie Hat

Repurpose actually taken into consideration considered one of your worn-out wool hats with a few hygge spirit! Making pom-poms is a laugh, however why prevent at one at the same time as you could make ten of them in various colorings? You and the whole circle of relatives can do this interest. You may also moreover even invite a few buddies along too.

What you'll need

•Needle and thread

•Yarn

•Scissors

•Cardboard

Instructions

1.   To make a bigger pom-pom, reduce out cardboard discs which is probably the same length.

2.   Each disc need to have a small hollow drilled through the middle earlier than being stacked. Make that the yarn can fit thru the hole.

three.   Holding the yarn in location collectively together with your fingers at the begin to prevent it from unraveling, loop it via the holes and all through the out of doors edges of the discs.

4.   Continue until the discs are absolutely and gently protected. Cut thru the yarn that surrounds the out of doors fringe of the card discs via putting the scissors a few of the cardboard discs.

5.   To bring together your pom-pom, carefully wrap a length of thread throughout the yarn within the space between the 2 discs, making sure to stable a knot on the stop. (Leave

enough thread to connect the pom-pom for your hat.)

6.   Cut the cardboard and cast off it from the pom-pom as soon as the yarn has firmly secured.

7.   To make your pom-pom exactly spherical, fluff it up and, if required, trim it with scissors.

8.   Put the pom-pom in your hat and stride into the brisk, chilly air with a cheery bounce.

Note: Use an entire lot of colourful yarns to create a pom-pom this is rainbow-hued. You can also purchase self-striping yarn, with the intention to carry out all of the be virtually right for you and supply your pom-pom a brighter appearance.

Felt slippers

The shoes of choice for pajama days want to be slippers. No slippers? No problem!

These felt slippers will keep your ft heat all year long. Show your toes some love.

You may also even deliver those to a chum or family member.

What you may need

•19.Five x 19.Five inch (50 x 50 cm) Felted wool square

•Scissors

•Chalk for dressmakers or fabric markers

•sturdy thread made of polyester or silk

•Darning needle, huge

•Paper

Instructions

1.     Use a photocopier to increase the template underneath in order that it's far two instances as huge and additional or lots less an inch longer than the simplest of your shoe before decreasing it out.

2.   Trace the template onto your felt, making sure that you lessen out the T shape with care.

three.   Sew the toe seam after folding the felt in 1/2 of lengthwise. You need to pinch the heel seams collectively. Sew from the top of the slipper to approximately 2 centimeters (three.Five inches) from the heel. Carefully snip into the heel to shape a small flap.

four.   This flap want to be securely stitched in location. Afterward, turn the slipper inner out and use your scissors to spherical the flap's edges for a completed look. You have options: save you there or fold the perimeters to the ankle and sew them to the slipper. Remember to expose the template, so the T is at the opportunity aspect whilst sewing the alternative slipper.

Note: The opportunities are infinite on the subject of which include more hygge. Consider along with lace, home made felt plants, pom-poms, or matching them in your chosen pajamas.

Lavender bags

Since historical instances, human beings have applied lavender for its healing advantages. Its aroma is calming and rejuvenating. Making lavender bags is simple, and they have masses of uses. Put one underneath your pillow to promote a restful night time time's sleep, or stash one in a drawer or cloth cupboard to preserve your clothes and bedding smelling clean.

When you are having a busy day, you may even bring one for your purse or pocket to help you unwind with its touchy fragrance.

What you could want

•Scissors

•Pins

•Pretty fabric (Your desire)

•Dried lavender

•Needle and thread

•Ribbon (Optional)

Instructions

1.    Measure the fabric and reduce out two rectangles which might be 6 thru 4.Five inches (16 x eleven.5 cm).

2.   With the patterned aspects going via each different, pin the two rectangles together.

three.    Sew across the rectangle, stopping approximately 34 inches (2 cm) from the alternative corner, starting midway down really certainly one of the fast facets.

4.   You can use the surrender of a pencil or a paintbrush to push out the corners, so they're pointed earlier than slicing off the corners and turning the rectangle the proper manner round on the identical time as pushing the cloth via the hole you have created.

five.   To make the seam at some point of the hole superb and directly, iron it.

6.   Fill with dried lavender (available online or from a nearby lavender farm); if you have get

proper of access to to a lavender bush, dry your private.

Note: Place a loop of ribbon halfway at some point of the pinnacle border of the distance in case you want to hang your bag up. Then, sew throughout the gap, backstitching over the ribbon to hold it in location.

# Chapter 4: Seasonal Outdoor/ Indoor Activities/Hobbies

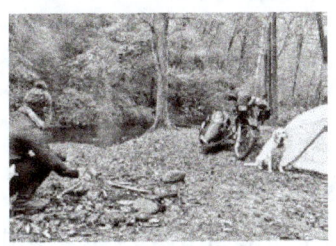

Hygge is greater than just staying warmness via the hearth and blockading out the bloodless. Whatever the weather, this economic disaster offers hints for purchasing the most out of nature and bonding with it via using indoor and outside sports or interests.

Natural Wonders

When It consists of Hygge and natural wonders, there are various sports, hobbies, and practices that you in all likelihood can do to reap a experience of enrichment. Doing so lets in us to get in touch with nature and our surroundings. This is splendid for experiencing the Hyggelig feeling.

Watching the sundown

Sunsets have a mystical and innately sturdy tremendous. These herbal marvels have moved poets and authors for millennia. We need to all take the time to recognize sunsets. Find a area with a view of the western horizon on a clean day. Prepare for the enjoy through dressing warmly and getting there early.

As the sun descends decrease within the sky, pink, orange, and gold colors start to shimmer. Sit with a pal or a cherished one and watch in delight. Regularly wearing out this conscious hobby or hobby is a smooth way to characteristic more wonder and beauty in your day.

Stargazing

The fantastic time to find out the marvels of the night time time time sky is on a smooth night time time.

A celebrity map and a couple of binoculars are all you want to appearance some incredible celestial items. For help in navigating the night time sky, get an night sky map from the Internet and buy or borrow a compass.

The best place for stargazing is a long way from towns and different slight-polluted regions; bear in mind going to a park, a hill, or a seaside. Find the North Star and stars in the Big Dipper, Orion, and Cassiopeia constellations. Watch out for meteors and some distance-off planets as properly. To preserve each adults and children glad even as stargazing, supply a blanket to put on, masses of warmth apparel, and a flask of warmth beverage. Perhaps even some small eats too.

Bonfires

The last out of doors hyggelig interest is building a bonfire. Organize a assembly with buddies and put together dinner over a campfire. Serve potatoes with butter after wrapping them in foil and burying them in the embers until the insides are fluffy and easy.

Make bonfire bananas, which is probably roasted bananas that have been reduce in 1/2 of lengthwise and full of chocolate chips, or roast marshmallows on lengthy sticks for dessert. As you gather round a roaring hearth, take a 2nd to lighten up and pleasure in the feeling of normal comfort and contentment.

How to assemble a bonfire

•Locate a secure spot far from homes, fences, wooden, shrubs, and rubbish or backyard waste.

•Create a small pit to location out the flames. It should be about 1 outside (1 meter) broader than you would like your fireside to be and about four inches (10 cm) deep.

•To preserve the hearth contained, surround the pit's area with bricks or large stones.

•Place a tinder bundle (wood shavings, newspaper, twigs, bark, grass, dry leaves, or maybe moss) on pinnacle of the firelighters within the center of the pit.

•To create a tepee shape, set up the dry kindling atop the tinder at forty five-degree angles, meeting in the center simply so the tinder also can gather oxygen and go away small areas within the kindling.

•Drop a lighted healthy in the tepee or area it underneath the tinder.

•When the kindling tepee collapses, add logs to feed the hearth.

•The tinder must ignite first, then the kindling.

•Make brilliant you really extinguish the fireside at night time's cease. Give yourself as a minimum 20 mins for this as it takes longer than you anticipate. When the hearth is cool, sell off some dirt or sand on pinnacle and spray water over it to extinguish the embers.

•Keep children a protracted way from the fireplace besides an person is looking them.

Toasting marshmallows within the the front of the hearth

Nothing is more hyggelig than toasted marshmallows, which is probably crisp at the outside and wonderfully mild at the inner. Place more than one marshmallows on the forestall of a kebab stick and take a seat down by means of manner of your fireplace or hearth pit to roast them till they flip golden to relive your formative years.

You can sandwich the marshmallow amongst graham crackers, or you can devour it complete. Keep damp wipes handy for any sticky fingers, and be careful due to the fact the deliciousness may be heated internal!

(A clean hyggelig hobby you can do with friends and own family; that once repeated enough can change into a totally unique interest.)

Fun In The Snow

Modest joys like waking as a whole lot because the number one frost of the one 12 months or, even higher, the primary snow fall are examples of small moments of Hygge. Casting the curtains exhibits a international covered with glistening, crystalline snow, this is in fact lovely. The simplest sound in the scene is the crunch of snow underfoot.

Long periods of silence in advance than the motion begins offevolved! Snow is an exceptional justification for appearing stupid and being a toddler all once more, having snowball battles, making snowmen, going sledding, and making snow angels. When the joyous shrieks and laughter have subsided, take the entire family for a walk at the identical time as you see how the environment have transformed proper right right into a wintry weather wonderland sparkling with snow and ice.

Once you have got got finished this and you have red cheeks and large smiles, return home in which you could experience warm liquids via the fireplace, a circle of relatives movie, and a head entire of fond reminiscences.

Woodland Walks

Wrap up, placed to your walking boots, and visit the woods to reconnect with the critical subjects in existence. Woods are extremely good places to appearance and concentrate for plants and fauna for the reason that timber offer safe haven for numerous species. You ought to probably pay attention an owl or cuckoo calling, look at fox or badger tracks, or every.

You may additionally even likely stumble upon a carpet of bluebells in the spring or discover tremendous conkers dispersed beneath the horse chestnut tree's branches within the fall. It's fun to find out the woods. There are such plenty of items to pick up and collect at some point of the experience, along with pine cones, leaves, acorns, and feathers, that you could flip them proper right into a scavenger hunt.

Hug a tree or balance on logs to embrace your playful side. It's a first rate technique to revitalize your self thru manner of spending time inside the woods. Trees supply forth chemical substances and aromas that enhance our mood and help us unwind. Go to the woods and take within the calming surroundings. Who is aware about, you may certainly have placed your new favored interest.

Bike Rides

Few matters offer you with a revel in of independence, like the use of a motorbike. It's a excellent low-effect fitness method that permits you to excite you as you freewheel down hills and motorcycle alongside tracks, just like you likely did while you have been a toddler. Enjoy the enjoyable warm temperature of the sun for your face and the breeze ruffling your hair.

While riding the pedals, stay in touch at the side of your body. There is not a extra thrilling manner to adventure for my part! And who is aware of, you may have definitely placed a brand new healthful hobby.

Picnics

Summer is the season most often related to picnics. Still, summer time furthermore has its drawbacks, which includes crunchy sand in your sandwiches, having to shoo curious animals away, and having to break out when an ominous little gray cloud will become a biblical downpour.

So why now not attempt a picnic inside the fall or winter while the climate is brighter? Food unites people, and no putting does it better than a picnic. A high-quality hyggelig experience is to percent food and chat at the same time as sitting on a blanket. Why now not plan a picnic wherein all of us brings a dish to percent?

Spread out severa blankets in a picturesque place, like a seaside, park, wooded place, or nature reserve; convey extra apparel in case it receives cool. Allow everyone to help themselves with notable cuisine on plates, then sit down and unwind. Picnics also may be spontaneous sports activities. You can take your dinner to the seashore, experience your lunch inside the park, or p.C. Some soup and flow into on a road adventure.

Enjoying the surroundings, food, and business company of others makes a picnic particular, no matter in which you are or with whom.

What's extra, you may flip picnicking into your very private personal interest; all you want is repetition.

Note: Keep in thoughts that a picnic does now not should be tough to be interesting. With warmth soup, chili, or stew in a flask, baked potatoes in foil, and heat chocolate and cookies for dessert, hold things sincere however cushty. Eating outdoors typically improves the taste of food!

Fruit Picking In The Hedgerows

Hedgerows in the autumn are bursting with mouthwatering secure to devour treasure; give up end result like elderberries and blackberries are begging to be picked. So acquire the untamed hedgerows in a bag or basket.

The whole own family can bond with nature at the same time as taking advantage of the rest of the satisfactory climate by means of the usage of going foraging. Pick mature elderberries in bunches to provide a lovable candy jelly, or gather sloes to make gin in a few areas—pluck blackberries from bushes to make a fruit crumble.

Always check to see if the goods you have foraged are constant to eat, so ensure to carry a guidebook or an expert. However, in case you spend a whole lot of time doing this, it's miles higher to name it what it's far—a hobby.

Winter Beach Walks

Winter coastal weather can supply sturdy winds, hard seas, and bitterly cold temperatures. Still, it additionally makes the seashore an interesting place for on foot, playing video video games, beachcombing, or simply taking component in being out of doors within the smooth air. Take a flask of a few factor warm and wrap up in competition to the cold.

Winter is one of the exceptional seasons for beachcombing because of the charming flotsam and jetsam that wintry weather storms produce. At low tide, stroll down and search the shingle for sharks' teeth. You can also moreover bring a kite, ball, and bat and make the maximum of the enough region to take satisfaction in an array of various sports sports or enjoy simply certainly one of your favourite interests.

Before leaving

•Check the tide instances, in particular if you intend to go to a section of the coast this is inaccessible at immoderate tide.

•Wear shoes with grips to prevent slipping on moist rocks or free shingles.

•Additionally, deliver a couple of binoculars if you take location to phrase a few coastal birds or a gray seal bobbing within the water.

## Chapter 5: Simple Pleasures

Hygge is ready appreciating the small matters

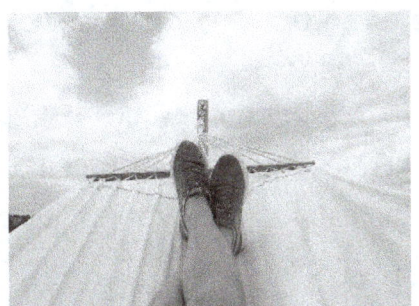

in lifestyles and taking the time to experience one's organization or some properly-earned "me time." For a day by day dose of Hygge, take the time to take satisfaction in the ones small pleasures and incorporate them into your lifestyles.

A Delightful Candle-lit Bath

One of the quickest strategies to go into a pleasing us of a of relaxation and entertainment is to take a warmth bath. Here's the way to make your relaxation room a chilled and healing spa retreat. Run your bathtub whilst along with a few bath salts to assist your muscle agencies.

Add more than one drops of virtually one of your preferred thrilling important oils, which includes lavender, neroli, or rose, to the water earlier than entering. Apply a face masks prepared from one mashed banana blended with a tablespoon of orange juice and a spoonful of honey to nourish your pores and pores and pores and skin.

Although it smells delicious enough to consume, resist the urge! The steam will then curl about you while you loosen up. Candles will add to the coziness. Step out of the tub, rinse your face with warmth water, and moisturize after soaking for round 20 mins.

Put on your coziest bathrobe, lighten up with a ebook or a cup of natural tea, and enjoy a well-earned snooze!

(It's first-class to combine the oil with some olive oil first; which incorporates critical oils right now to hot water reasons them to evaporate, fast reducing recuperation advantages.)

Reading By The Fireplace

What is probably greater leisurely than analyzing an super ebook in the the front of a roaring hearth at the same time as paying attention to the rain patter at the window? Spend some time studying a ghost tale, playing a thriller, or rereading some antique favorites.

Try reading aloud to a completely unique someone on the identical time as the hearth flickers softly in the historical past. It's the appropriate entertainment interest to interact in on a darkish, bloodless day or a dark wintry weather night time time.

Partake In A Feel-Good Movie

Watching a sense-accurate movie whilst curled below a blanket or cover is one of the best methods to beautify your temper. The following movies are positive to make your day higher, whether or not or now not you watch them by way of your self or collectively with your circle of relatives at the couch at the identical time as retaining popcorn and drinks.

Top ten revel in-proper movies: (My Opinion)

1. Forrest Gump

2. Ferris Bueller's Day Off

3. Back To The Future

4. The Shawshank Redemption

5. Amélie

6. Little Miss Sunshine

7. Dirty Dancing

8. Groundhog Day

9. It's A Wonderful Life

10. Pretty Women

Top ten family movies: (My Opinion)

1.  Any traditional Walt Disney film (e.G., Cinderella, Snow White and the seven dwarfs, Pinocchio)

2.  Wallace & Gromit: The Curse Of The Were-Rabbit

three.  Beauty and the Beast

4.  Toy Story

five.  E.T. The Extra-Terrestrial

6.  The Goonies

7.  Up

8.  Shrek

9.  Frozen

10. Ratatouille

Playing Games With Family And Friends

Find your desired leisure board video games in the attic and supply them a excellent cleaning. Playing video video games along with your circle of relatives through way of manner of the hearth also can make even the most depressing day interesting. Pass out pieces of home made cake, mulled wine, and freshly brewed coffee.

Connecting with the humans for your existence while having amusing is the number one motive of hyggelig recreation-gambling. Try your hand at a traditional recreation like Jenga or Scrabble to appearance how agile you are physical and mentally.

Hygge Playlist

The sound of burning wooden, the patter of rain on glass, and the crisp flick of pages moving all have loads to recommend, but the ones aren't the simplest sounds that deliver Hygge. Searching through your song library won't take prolonged to find out songs that assist you to find out the Scandinavian idea.

Some tunes represent the loosen up of the outside air, the hug of a cherished one, and nights of introspective peace and pleasure. You can find out a hyggelig music on masses of your favorite albums, whether or now not it is blues and u.S., indie, jazz, soul, or a few difficulty style lighting fixtures your hygge flame.

You can use your hygge playlist as the first-rate records music for diverse pursuits, sports activities, or hobbies, or you can actually lean decrease once more, close to your eyes, and glide at the melodic eddies at the identical time as you enjoy a few masses-needed enjoyment time.

Company

Self-hygge is feasible. Hyggeligt consists of diverse sports activities, which incorporates cuddling up below a blanket along aspect your preferred TV display on a wet Sunday afternoon, sipping red wine at the same time as looking a rainstorm, or without a doubt sitting via the window and taking in the environment.

However, the most funny instances continually seem like shared with others. My father and his brothers nowadays celebrated their fiftieth birthdays, in order that they hired a giant summer time cabin on Denmark's west coast and invited certainly anyone. Sand dunes surrounded the cabin, that have turn out to be placed in a rugged, barren vicinity wherein the wind commonly blows brutally.

There, we did no longer something but eat, drink, chat, and walk down the seashore for an entire weekend. That have become, in my view, the coziest and most leisurely weekend I had that one year.

Casualness

The majority of hyggelige moments seem like built on a basis of leisure or laxness. You should be cushty in order for you and your internet site website traffic to Hygge. There isn't any want to formalize whatever. Come as you are and act thus.

For instance, I participated in a Champagne grape harvest one fall. I visited the place a few years in the past with 3 pals, and we decided to go to the Marquette winery, wherein I had previously labored. A hyggelig afternoon become spent within the winery and in the rustic rural kitchen.

It had a low ceiling and flagstone floors, where we had been delivered to Glennie, the female of the house, and her son, who, by means of this time, have become an grownup. Even even though I hadn't seen Glennie and her toddler in some time, there was no want for formality due to the fact the environment modified into informal and laid-lower back.

You also can experience a casual come across with the aid of way of the use of journeying someplace new with near friends or family, so why now not flow out of your consolation region?

Get Closer To Nature

Being in nature lets in you to permit your defend down and gives a certain simplicity, whether or not or not sitting thru a river in Sweden, a winery in France, or simply in your garden or a close-by park. When we are near nature, we are not preoccupied with amusing gadgets or juggling various picks.

There is extraordinary amazing enterprise and awesome discussion, no more or luxury. A brief way to Hygge is to apply smooth, leisurely, rustic additives.

Being In The Present Moment

Being located in memorable moments has a detail to play. Hygge is characterized through a massive focus on experiencing and appreciating the present second. Every summer time, my extraordinary buddy, his father, and I would circulate sailing.

There modified into nowhere else we needed to be all through that tenting trip. We weren't associated. No phone, No electronic mail. We have to unwind and experience the event due to the reality we were surrounded thru nature and notable organisation agency.

I understand a few matters more than being at the helm because the music blasts under deck under complete white sails and a blue sky. The additives of these trips in which we have been docked in the harbors we visited had been the maximum amusing. Every night time time after dinner, everyone sat on the deck to have a look at the sun skip down even as gambling our put up-dinner Irish coffees and taking note of the wind within the deliver's sails. Hygge is that.

Utilizing some of the components referred to in advance can be the high-quality manner to create hygge memories. Occasionally, you is probably able to in shape every object into the pot. That occurs for me in excursion cabins. In many respects, living in a cabin gives all the aforementioned blessings. Many of my finest youth enjoyment reminiscences revolve spherical a small summer season cabin we used to rent for my family each year, about six miles outside of the town from May to September.

My brother and I might also need to take satisfaction in the in no manner-ending summer time days while even the night time time became without darkness at that aspect of 365 days. We may also need to play soccer, adventure bicycles, find out tunnels, climb wood, entice fish, create dams and forts, sleep in tree huts, and hide beneath boats on the beach—all within the spirit of Hygge and enjoyment.

Savor And Be Grateful for The Moment

Savoring is usually about thankfulness. It is set appreciating the existing and the honest joys of delectable delicacies and amazing organisation. It is paying proper interest to the whipped cream-crowned heat chocolate. Simply positioned, Hygge is all about residing within the present and making the maximum indulging in leisurely moments.

We regularly nag every different to no longer take some thing as a right. When you get a gift, saying "thank you" isn't sufficient to specific gratitude. It consists of remembering that you are living within the now, permitting yourself to apprehend your life as it's miles, and that specialize in all you've got in preference to all you lack. Clichés?

Totally. We are, unfortunately, keen to comply to new things and sports, in particular super ones, due to the truth our emotional system enjoys novelty. As a prevent stop end result, you must don't forget glowing motives to precise gratitude in preference to letting your mind wander to the identical antique mind.

Studies claim that feeling grateful encourages human beings to stand lower once more and understand what they've got extra and decreases the threat that they will take it as a right. Because Hygge is commonly approximately relishing small joys, it could help us enjoy appreciative of the regular.

Hygge is maximizing the prevailing, however it's also a method for making prepared for and keeping enjoyment through smooth enjoyment sports activities or pastimes. Because of this, Hygge might be one of the reasons for why Danes always document excessive stages of happiness. In addition to having guidelines that assure them time to find out big connections.

Danes charge spending time with their families and pals and cultivating lasting relationships.

Hygge During Office Hours

Hygge, but, is not pretty much curling up on your hyggekrog at home in the front of the fireside, eating Irish coffees on the deck, or taking thing in snug cottages. The Danish count on that Hygge can—and should—get up at paintings. So how could probably place of job hours be made cozier or greater leisurely? Well, obviously, cakes and candles.

But this is best the start. Consider how you could make topics greater informal, comfortable, and egalitarian. Here are 5 pointers to encourage Hygge within the place of business.

Five easy Hyggelig activities

1.  Organize A Potluck Friday: Why now not plan potlucks for lunch at some point every week in region of packing a lunch for your self? Everyone feels hygge after they percent.

2.  Set Up An Office Garden: You can growth the Hygge through along with some vegetation if the workspace or the surroundings allow it. It might be an exquisite method to lessen strain thru giving them a bit attention every day. If you plant vegetables you could devour for lunch, you get bonus factors for Hygge.

3.  Bring Your Dog To Work: This is an extraordinary manner to growth productiveness by way of manner of putting

timed goals to offer the fluffy one a miles-favored belly rub for you and them.

four.   Try To Make The Office More Homely: Ask your manager if they might perhaps set up a few couches for people to apply once they need to do a quick-casual assembly or have lengthy papers to examine.

5.   Hygge Cubicle Life: Perhaps you are not capable of regulate the administrative center, however what approximately your desk? Would it's miles possible to feature some flora and preserve a few cushty socks within the drawer for working in the evenings? You may moreover take it a step further and envision your workspace due to the fact the Batcave of Hygge, turning into the unsung hygge hero. At the same time, your coworkers are eating lunch, the simplest who leaves a delicious piece of chocolate on their desks.

A Simple Leisure Itinerary From Jan To Dec

Some human beings receive as real with the weather in Denmark is unhappy, windy, and damp; others declare there are remarkable winters, one grey and one inexperienced. It want to be no surprise that Danes spend most in their time indoors in some unspecified time in the future of the wintry climate, given the climate.

Most Danes try to spend as an awful lot time outdoor as they're capable of for the duration of the summer season inside the vain preference of absorbing a few solar, but from November to March, the weather drives Danes to stay indoors.

All Danes have left to do in the path of the wintry climate is hygge at home as they can't participate in iciness sports activities activities in their usa like Sweden and Norway or revel in time outdoor like in southern Europe.

January: Movie night

A casual movie night time time with friends and own family is the proper way to unwind in January. Allow certainly every body to supply food to proportion, and choose out an vintage traditional you have got all watched. This manner, it won't rely loads if parents speak a little in the course of the movie. Finding the fastest technique to summarize the plot of the chosen film is a fun addition to movie night time.

The Lord of the Rings trilogy and Forrest Gump have become "Drug-addicted girls take benefit of a mentally handicapped boy for many years" and "Group spends nine hours returning jewelry," respectively.

February: Ski revel in

Plan a revel in to the mountains presently of yr in conjunction with your buddies and family when you have the danger. The maximum notable part of the ski enjoy is the Hygge, no matter the breathtaking mountain perspectives, interesting slope speeds, and great air top notch.

The magic occurs whilst you, your buddies, and your circle of relatives go back in your cabin after an extended day on the slopes to unwind with espresso in peace. Don't forget about approximately approximately to deliver the Grand Marnier!

March: Theme month

This is probably a technique to jumpstart the Hygge in case you and your own family are planning a summer time tour. Spend March doing a digital tour of Spain if you're heading there. To get a head begin at the language, I mean "exploring" via looking Spanish movies, cooking tapas, and, if you have youngsters, perhaps spending one night time writing Post-its in Spanish on the chairs (sillas), desk (mesa), and plates (platos).

If you are not going on excursion this 12 months, you could pick out out your dream location or use a topic from a state you have got previously visited (get out the photograph albums). Bring america domestic in case you can't adventure there.

April: Hiking and cooking over an open fireplace

April can be an incredible month for individuals who experience paddling, hiking, and tenting. Weather-smart, it is probably a touch cold, so don't forget to maintain the ones woolen socks (they're warm), however the month has blessings due to the reality there are fewer mosquitoes.

Without Wi-Fi, "What the hell are we going to do out right here?" Your heart charge and strain degrees will decrease whilst you get via this. Hiking is a hygge Easter egg because it promotes slowness, rusticity, and community.

The cuisine might be organized, simmered over the fireplace at the identical time as you acquire wooden for the fireplace, and then loved along with your friends at the identical time as sipping whiskey out of doors after dinner. If you are going someplace for Easter, recollect to bring the chocolate eggs for the children.

May: Weekend cabin

May is the first rate month to start the use of the geographical place due to the truth the times are growing longer; which means there is more time for amusement and interests. The greater primitive the cabin, the more hygge; likely considered one of your friends has get admission to to as a minimum one, or you may discover an inexpensive condominium.

An introduced gain is a fire. Pack a few board video video games for gloomy days. May weekends can also provide the primary hazard to have a BBQ. Nothing like putting out with the resource of the grill with a lager on your hand for summer hygge.

June: The summer time solstice and elderflower cordial

Elderflowers can be harvested early June and used to make cordial or lemonade.

On June 23, St. John's Eve, Danes have a take a look at the summer season solstice. My favourite custom is this one. In Denmark, the solar units in June at 11 p.M. On a night time time that in no way absolutely is going darkish.

As the sun starts offevolved to slowly set, there can be a bittersweet popularity that the instances gets shorter the next day, and we're able to begin the prolonged ascent into darkness. This might be the right night time time for a picnic. Gather your loved ones and ignite a bonfire.

(Because of the mild, they will be typically lit quite past due; in case you need to occupy the kids on the same time as you wait, that is a superb occasion for an egg-and-spoon race.)

Elderflower cordial

This elderflower cordial will fragrance of summer season whether or no longer you drink it warm temperature in the wintry weather or cold on a warm summer season day. Additionally, your house will fragrance like summer time hygge at the same time as you make the cordial by using manner of leaving the flora and lemons in a pan for twenty-4 hours. Just one sniff proper away takes me decrease back to the summers I spent as a toddler.

Ingredients

•30 clusters of elderflowers

•3 huge lemons

•6 glasses of water (forty eight ounces., 1.2L)

•8 cups of sugar (1610g, sixty four ounces)

Instructions

1. Place the elderflower clusters in a massive dish after very well washing them.

2.    Slice the lemons, scrub them in heat water, after which add them to the bowl's clusters.

3.   Add the sugar after bringing the water to a boil.

4.    Add the boiling water to the basin maintaining the lemon segments and elderflower clusters.

five.    Place a lid on the bowl and allow the lemonade to sit down for 3 days.

6.   Pour the liquid into bottles after straining it. Put it in the refrigerator to calm down and serve whilst ready.

July: Summer picnic


Danes recognize spending time outdoor in July. The evenings are nevertheless long, and the weather is warmness. This time of 365 days is proper for a picnic in a park, on a meadow, or through the ocean. Those are some options but go away the city out. Invite your family, friends, friends, or inexperienced persons down the road.

Make it a potluck amassing so that everyone brings something to provide. Because they are greater egalitarian, potluck dinners are normally cozier. They emphasize sharing food in addition to responsibilities and obligations.

August: The perseid meteor bathe

For a starry night time, convey blankets. Although the mild nights proper now of twelve months might not be perfect for stargazing, the Perseid meteor shower is to be had in mid-August, commonly accomplishing its top activity from August eleven to 13th. With Andromeda to the east and Cassiopeia to the north, maintain an eye fixed constant out for the Perseus constellation within the northeast.

Bring a ebook of Greek mythology recollections for your youngsters to have a look at whilst you expect the taking pix stars if you have any. The Eta Aquarid meteor bathe is viable for humans in the southern hemisphere. It generally reaches its height in late April or early May.

September: Mushroom foraging

Although they may be determined beginning in late summer time, mushrooms greater regularly than now not seem in the autumn. The meals you have grown, caught, or foraged yourself has the fantastic taste and a immoderate hygge element.

Invite loved ones along for a foraging adventure within the wild. Find an expert mushroom forager and ask them to accompany you on a forage. This might be counseled because of the reality consuming the incorrect mushrooms may be deadly. Many towns offer organization excursions.

October: chestnuts

It's time for chestnuts. Take your children's chestnut-looking and use the nuts to carve figures of animals. Buy safe to eat chestnuts for the grownups, lessen a pass within the pointy give up with a knife, and roast them at two hundred ranges Fahrenheit (98 tiers Celsius) for approximately half-hour, or until the skins open and the interiors are gentle.

Add a few butter and salt after casting off the difficult outer skin. Pick buy some mandarins, roasted chestnuts, and a replica of Hemingway's A Moveable Feast if you simply need a few hygge time to your self. It takes vicinity in Paris within the Twenties even as Hemingway became a suffering author.

November: Soup prepare dinner dinner-off

Winter is on its manner. It's time to find out new soup recipes and dig out the vintage ones. Invite cherished ones and probable a few friends over for a soup competition. Everyone contributes elements to make a unmarried-man or woman soup. Prepare many small soup servings for everybody to pattern, taking turns.

My move-to recipe is a pumpkin-ginger soup, that is wonderful with a chunk of crème fraîche. Baking some home made bread is a few thing more you can do as the host. Hygge is simply present while bread is freshly organized.

December: ÆBLESKIVER and GLØGG (Pancake Puffs)

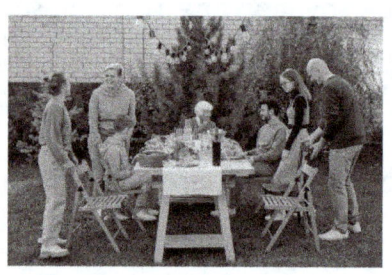

# Chapter 6: Comforting Recipes For Cozy Nights In

Hygge is all about having a laugh with the humans you care approximately, and one of the most proper techniques to perform this is to acquire for a meal or tea and cake and communicate approximately the vital (and unimportant) things in lifestyles. Food hugs, and it heals. The following recipes will assist offer hygge happiness right away.

You Are What You Eat

I accept as real with Alice Waters might be hygge if Hygge have been someone. She indicates many of the essential traits of Hygge with a cushty, unhurried, and leisurely way of residing. She also appears to understand the importance of brilliant, hearty meals within the employer of pleasant human beings. In present day years, there was loads of interest in new Nordic cuisine.

Noma, which debuted in 2003 and has been named the maximum splendid eating place inside the world 4 instances because 2010, has been the center of hobby. Even if a dish of live shrimp blanketed in ants might also take keep of hobby, it is not an ordinary Danish dish. An low fee version of the traditional Danish lunch dish, smorrebrod, or open-faced sandwiches on rye bread with pickled herring or leverpostej (liver paste—a spreadable concoction of baked, chopped pig's liver and lard), is served.

You want to be wondering that those ants are beginning to appearance tasty. A conventional Danish cookbook with the name 50 Shades of Meat and Potatoes might be suitable for dinner. The common Dane consumes 100 and five pounds of meat every year, with beef being the most famous meat in the u . S ..

Hygge is in element related to the excessive degrees of meat, candies, and coffee consumption in Denmark. Giving yourself a address and a vacation from the trials of healthy living are every crucial additives of the hygge manner of life. Sweets are scrumptious; a cake is cozily comfortable; each coffee and heat chocolate are leisurely and thrilling.

Not a lot with carrot sticks. The hygge ritual continuously consists of a few issue depraved. However, it should not be some element excessive or fancy. Foie gras isn't cozily cushty. Yet a warming stew, greater so if all of us consume from the same bowl.

Hot Drinks

Eighty-six percentage of Danes consider that Hygge is related to heat drinks. The Danes' desired hot beverage is espresso. However, they also revel in tea, warm chocolate, and mulled wine. You likely already understand how plenty the Danes experience their espresso if you're eager on Danish TV dramas like Borgen or The Killing. There is hardly ever a state of affairs this is going through without someone getting espresso, making coffee, or asking a person else, "Coffee?" Danish humans drink approximately 33 percentage more coffee in keeping with capita than Americans.

The Danish language makes specific the relationship among espresso and Hygge. Another compound phrase that mixes Hygge and coffee is kaffe hygge, that is widely used. "Come to kaffe hygge," together with "kaffe hygge and cake," "kaffe hygge and exercise," and "kaffe hygge and knitting."

There is kaffe Hygge everywhere. Even kaffe Hygge has a net web page that encourages customers to "Live life nowadays like there's no espresso tomorrow." So at the same time as you may gain Hygge with out espresso, it virtually allows. Holding a pleasing heat cup of coffee on your palms has a calming effect. Hygge can virtually flourish right right here.

Iced Vanilla Cookies

As they bake, the ones delicious cookies will fill your property with the outstanding heady scent of vanilla. They are warm, gooey, and buttery proper out of the oven—the right melt-in-your-mouth dessert to serve site visitors.

(Produces kind of 24 cookies)

Ingredients

•9¾ oz., (275g) Unsalted butter

•1 Teaspoon, zero.1 oz (4.9g) Vanilla extract

•1 Medium egg, lightly overwhelmed

•3½ oz. (100g) Superfine granulated sugar

•3½ oz. (100g) Unsalted butter

To beautify

•2-three Drops of meals coloring (Your preference)

•three-four Tablespoons, 2 ounces (0.05L) water

•14 ounces (400g) Powdered sugar

Method

1.   Set the oven's temperature to 375°F (a hundred 90°C, Gas five).

2.   In a bowl, combine the butter and sugar via manner of beating them collectively.

3.   Adding a chunk at a time, beat in the egg and vanilla extract.

four.   Add the flour and stir till a dough office work.

5.   Roll the dough to a thickness of 34 inches on a piece ground lightly dusted with flour (1 cm).

6.   Using cookie cutters, make cookies from the dough and area them on a baking sheet organized with parchment paper.

7.   Cookies need to be baked till golden brown (spherical 8–10 minutes).

8.   Transfer to a cord rack after allowing it to harden for 5 mins. Make the icing on the same time as the cookies are cooling.

9.   As directed on the packet, sift the powdered sugar into a big mixing bowl and add the water, stirring till the mixture is easy.

10. Use a knife to effortlessly spread the icing onto the cookies and a piping bag to function decorations. Stir within the food coloring.

11. Place aside until the icing becomes strong, and serve while organized.

Cinnamon Hot Chocolate

Indulgent heat chocolate is probably hygge if it had been a beverage. This decadent heat chocolate recipe is kind of a comfortable embrace in a cup. Whether on a moist day or a cold winter afternoon, I'm effective you can enjoy this warm chocolate as an entire lot as I do.

(Serves one)

Ingredients

•2 Tablespoons, 1 ounces (28.3g), and (180ml)/(6 oz.) milk (dairy or nut)

•½ Teaspoon, zero.08 ounces. (2.84g) vanilla extract

•¼ Teaspoon, zero.04 ounces (1.42g) floor cinnamon

•1 Tablespoon, 0.Five oz. (17.7g) sugar

•1 Tablespoon, 0.05 ounces. (17.7g) cocoa powder

To serve (Optional)

•Cinnamon

•Marshmallows

•Cream

Method

1.    Mix the cocoa powder, sugar, milk, cinnamon, and vanilla in a mug.

2.   As quickly due to the fact the aggregate resembles a thick syrup, stir it with a fork or a piece whisk.

3.   Warm the very last milk over medium warm temperature until it starts to boil, then pour it into the mug with the chocolate syrup and carefully whisk.

four.   Serve with a sprinkling of cinnamon and a dollop of cream or marshmallows for extra decadence.

Roasted Chestnuts

The best justification for spending time together with your circle of relatives thru the fireside is roasting chestnuts. When cooked to perfection, their faded interiors turn nutty, creamy, and fairly candy. Serve them undeniable or with melted butter that has been pro.

(Serves 4-6)

Ingredients

•2¼ lbs (1kg) Chestnut

For the spiced butter

•Pinch of nutmeg, salt, and sugar

•1 Cinnamon stick

•2 ounces (60g) Unsalted butter

Method

1.    Achieve a temperature of 4 hundred°F (two hundred°C, Gas 6).

2.   When roasting the chestnuts, you need to make an prolonged slit or a pass inside the curving shell via way of using a sharp knife to place them on their flat factors. They can flee with out detonating).

three.    Place in a unmarried layer, flat-side down, on a roasting pan, and bake till the pores and skin tears apart. It need to take about half of-hour. Peel the difficult pores and pores and pores and skin from the chestnuts after they're cold sufficient to address. Take the sweet, white kernel out of its pores and pores and skin and placed it in your mouth.

Method to bake on the fireplace

1.  In a solid iron frying pan or skillet, set up the prepared chestnuts in a unmarried layer.

2.  Place the pan internal the hearth's burning embers.

three.  To make certain same cooking, flip the chestnuts now and again. Cooking them will take 5 to 10 mins

Instructions for the spiced butter

1.  Spices, salt, and sugar are added after the butter has been melted over low warmth.

2.  Take off the cinnamon stick after the combination has melted, then pour it right right into a small bowl for dipping.

Berry Jam

Making your jam is simply one example of the tiny topics that make Hygge attractive. The berries are grow to be jars of scrumptious loveliness after an hour spent stirring, bottling, and labeling inside the kitchen. These jars are actually ready to be spread on warmness toast or scones.

Sticky and sweet, this jam will make you feel heat and satisfied indoors via growing something with the useful resource of hand. Pick your berries for jam for the happiest Hygge!

(Produces small jars)

Ingredients

•17 ½ oz9500g) Mixed seasonal berries

•1 ½ (zero.Seventy five oz) Tablespoons of lemon juice

•10 ½ oz. (300g) Sugar

Method

1. The berries must be installed a massive pot, slowly delivered to a boil, and then simmered for five mins.

2. After including the sugar, stir the mixture for 10 to 15 mins. Add the lemon juice after taking the pan off the warm temperature.

3. Fill sterilized jars with the jam, then cowl with a lid.

four. Allow to sit back and set. If saved in a groovy, dry pantry, the jam will final for at the least a twelve months, but as soon as opened, it wants to be stored inside the refrigerator.

Gingerbread House

Few subjects better capture the magic of Christmas than a gingerbread domestic, this is why Christmas is the height hygge season. Even even though building a gingerbread house takes time, the whole own family may be engrossed for hours, and children will revel in the use of their creativity to beautify the house with snowy frosting and treats.

(Builds one house)

Ingredients

•Unsalted butter, one hundred 75 grams, or six ¼ ounces.

•7.Five ounces (2 hundred g) smooth, mild-brown sugar

•1 ½ tbsp, 0.Seventy five ounceslemon juice, and one teaspoon, zero.1 ounces (four.9g) lemon zest

•five oz. Of liquid (one hundred fifty g) molasses

•2 Beaten eggs

•thirteen ¼ oz. (375 g) smooth flour

•Two teaspoons of baking powder, 28.3g (zero.Nine oz.)

•1 Tablespoon 17.7g (0.5 oz) ginger root

•Ground allspice, two teaspoons 10g (0.35 oz.)

For The Icing

•Egg whites, six

•3¾ kilos (1.Seventy five kg) (1.Seventy 5 kg) sprinkled with sugar powder

•Various sweets for adorning, collectively with gum drops, licorice cubes, small fruit snacks, white chocolate buttons (roof tiles), and colored sprinkles

Method

1.      Cut out bureaucracy from skinny cardboard to use as templates for the residence's partitions and roof. You'll want a triangle gable, a roof rectangle, a aspect wall (four.Seventy five x 7.Seventy 5 inches)(12cm x 19cm), an give up wall (four.Seventy five x 5 inches)(12cm x 12cm), and a triangular gable (four.Seventy 5 x 3 x three inches)(12cm x 7.5cm x 7.5cm) and a roof rectangle

(four.Seventy five x nine inches)(12cm x 23cm).

2.    Tape collectively the four.Seventy five-inch-lengthy triangular gable piece's lengthy difficulty and one of the 4.Seventy 5-inch facets of the give up wall.

3.   Incorporate the butter and sugar together until they will be slight and frothy to create the gingerbread combination. Lemon juice, zest, and molasses need to all be brought. Incorporate  beaten eggs. To create a dough, sift the flour, baking powder, and spices into the combination. The dough on parchment paper, then located it inside the refrigerator. Six portions of dough must be created, with being significantly large than the others. On a ground that has been gently dusted with flour, roll out the 4 smaller portions, and then lessen out two component walls and  give up walls with triangular gables (see predicted measurements above). Cut out  roof portions from the last dough by means of manner of way of rolling them out.

4.   The gingerbread forms need to be placed on organized baking sheets and baked for 10 minutes at 375°F (one hundred ninety°C, Gas five) or till crisp.

five.   Take out of the oven and allow cool for some time. Transfer to twine racks, and go away to harden in a unmarried day. You ought to lightly whisk  egg whites to make the icing, then gradually upload one-1/3 of the powdered sugar till the mixture is simple and paperwork company peaks. You can now begin building the house. One of the aspect partitions want to be firmly pressed into the nine-inch line of icing that has been unfold or piped onto the cake board to ensure that it sits upright. To provide the wall extra balance, you will possibly need to channel a chunk bit more icing down each factor of it. Ice the detail edges of an stop wall on each factors. Spread or pipe an icing line parallel to the primary wall at the board, and then push the forestall wall firmly into the icing. To create the walls of your private home, repeat this approach with the last aspect and forestall walls. Before the use of, permit the floor harden for as a minimum  hours.

For the roof

1.   Pipe or spread a relatively thick layer of icing on top of all of the walls to characteristic the inspiration for the roof. Then, press the roof quantities into the icing, making sure the roof overflows the partitions to shape the eaves.

2.   You can be part of the two roof components with the aid of manner of way of piping or making use of a few icing along the roof's crest. Leave to harden in a unmarried day.

three.   You can now get started out on making a few frosting to enhance your house. Four egg whites are gently whipped, then the last powdered sugar is brought.

4.  To make doorways, home home windows, and roof tiles for the residence, use icing to stick fantastic chocolates to the form. Add

icing to the roof to make snow, then pinnacle with icing sugar.

Fruit Crumble

Fruit fall apart cooked from scratch is the suitable comfort food that lets in you to prevent the flu. This apple and blackberry crumble has a thick, golden oaty topping for a delicious crunch and is flavored with cinnamon. Serve it with dollops of custard or ice cream.

(Serves 4)

Ingredients

•5 Apples, cubed after being peeled

•a hundred fifty g or 5 ¼ ouncesof blackberries

•6 Tablespoons, 85g (three oz.) moderate mild-brown sugar

•½ Teaspoon 2.84g (0.05 oz..) cinnamon

•Vanilla extract, 1 teaspoon four.9g (0.1 ounces)

For the topping

•100g (three ½ oz.) of ordinary flour

•Cinnamon and  tablespoons of brown sugar

•Unsalted butter, chilled and cubed, 1 ¾ oz. (50 g).

•four Tablespoons, 56.7g (2 oz.) of oats

Method

1.   Set the oven's temperature to 350°F (100 80°C, Gas four).

2.   Combine the diced apples, blackberries, sugar, cinnamon, and vanilla essence in a heavy-bottomed pot.

three.   Mix very well, then prepare dinner for five mins over medium heat.

four.   Making the topping inside the period in-between consists of combining the flour, sugar, and cinnamon in a small bowl.

5.  Oats are introduced after the aggregate has been rubbed with butter till it resembles breadcrumbs.

6.  After spooning it into the ovenproof dish, region the disintegrate on the fruit mixture— Bake for 15 to twenty mins, or till bubbling and brown.

Hot Spiced Fruit Punch

Hygge is all about playing lifestyles with the humans you love, enjoyable in the front of a hearth, and possibly clinking glasses as they are packed with some thing heat and delectable. This recipe combines unusual spices with wintry climate give up stop result and is sort of a cushty embody in a cup.

(Serves 6-8)

Ingredients

•Orange one

•10 Whole cloves

•Choose severa juices, consisting of orange, crimson grape, pineapple, apple, and cranberry, for your five liters (169 oz..) of unsweetened fruit juice.

•250 ml (eight.Four ounces) or 1 cup of water

•¼ Teaspoon 2.84g (0.05 oz..) floor cinnamon

•¼ Teaspoon 2.84g (zero.05 oz...) ground nutmeg

•1 Stick of cinnamon (plus more to serve)

•Star anise, one (plus more to serve)

•1 apple

•A small amount of cranberries

•Lemon juice from one freshly squeezed lemon

Method

1.   Push the cloves into the peel of one half of of of the orange after slicing it in half of.

2.     Fill a saucepan alongside facet your combination of fruit juices totaling one liter.

3.  Then use a timber spoon to mix inside the cinnamon and nutmeg powders.

4.  Add the pan collectively with half of of of the orange filled with cloves.

five.  The famous person anise and cinnamon stick.

6.  On a selection, warm the mixture and permit it to simmer for 20 minutes.

7.  Through a sieve, pour the mixture from the pan right into a basin and then proper right into a bowl.

8.  In the strainer, throw out the orange and the complete spices.

nine.  Slice the apple and the other 1/2 of of the orange. Include the slices inside the bowl along aspect the cranberries and lemon juice.

10. Punch need to be poured into a tumbler the usage of a jug or a ladle. Now mild the fireplace, take within the icy vista out of doors, take a seat down decrease again, and unwind.

## Mulled Wine

It splendid desires a couple of minutes to make and is effective to heat you from the indoors. This is a outstanding seasonal birthday celebration drink, manner to the intoxicating spice perfume. This drink will assist with offering an uplifting ecosystem for you and your buddies/own family.

(Serves eight)

Ingredients

•A bottle of purple wine bottle

•1 Quartered orange

•2 Ounces (60 g) of brown sugar or demerara

•1 Stick of cinnamon

•Grated nutmeg, one teaspoon four.9g (zero.1 oz)

•Fresh bay leaf, one

•Two complete cloves

•Star anise,

To serve (Optional)

•Orange slices with cloves on them

•One stick of cinnamon

•Anise famous individual

Method

1.   You should add one-fourth of the purple wine to a saucepan.

2.   Add the spices, demerara, brown sugar, and orange slices after stirring.

three.   Once the sugar has dissolved, boil gently.

4.   Add extra sugar or spices to taste after tasting for sweetness and spice.

5.   The mixture should begin to resemble syrup after being added to a boil for a few minutes to allow the spices to permeate.

6.   Reduce the warmth to a low setting, stir in the final wine and movie star anise, and cook

dinner dinner dinner for a couple of minutes—strain into mugs or glasses that are heatproof.

7.    Serve with orange slices decorated with clove, cinnamon, and large name anise if you need it even warmer.

Mulled Cider

Mulled cider is the proper beverage for gloomy days and cold nights spent via manner of the hearth. It now not handiest makes your kitchen scent like a candle save, but it additionally makes you enjoy higher. Impossible to stand as a great deal as with its citrus, rum, clove, and apple flavors, this cider recipe is a super manner to deplete windfall apples.

(Serves 8)

Ingredients

•8 cups (2 liters) (sixty seven ounces) cider

- Two apples studded with cloves

- Four cinnamon sticks

- Five complete allspice berries

- Zest of 1 orange

- Two measures of rum (darkish is fine)

To serve (Optional)

- Star anise

- Slices of apples

- Cinnamon sticks

Method

1.  In a massive saucepan, contain all the materials and warmth to a mild simmer for half-hour.

2.  Take care to make certain that it does no longer boil.

3.  Turn off the heat, strain, and pour into heatproof glasses or mugs after moving the liquid to a heatproof basin.

four.   Serve with cinnamon sticks, famous character anise, and apple slices.

Butternut Squash Soup

Make a hearty cup of creamy butternut squash soup to welcome your self home. This dinnertime delicacy is the nutritional same of a snug knit sweater and is simple to make (plus, you could reheat it for lunch!).

(Serves 2)

Ingredients

•2 Tiny or one big butternut squash

•A few freshly-chopped, easy sage leaves

•Black pepper freshly ground

•1 to 2 Tablespoons (14.3g/28.3g)(zero.Five ounces1 ounces.) of olive oil

•2 Chopped onions

•1(1 liter)(34 oz...) of vegetable or bird inventory

To serve (Optional)

•Crème fraîche

•Pumpkin seeds

•Fresh thyme leaves sprinkled on pinnacle

•Blue cheese fragment

•Both salt and pepper

Method

1.   Set the oven's temperature to 350°F (100 eighty°C, Gas four).

2.   Remove the seeds from the butternut squash without peeling it, then reduce it into massive pieces. Combine with the black pepper, olive oil, and sage leaves. Put the aggregate in a roasting pan and prepare dinner it for 35 to forty five minutes.

3.   In a extremely good pot, saute the onions until they may be apparent at the same time as the squash is cooking. Add the combination to the onions and cowl with stock once the butternut squash has softened and the sage

leaves have come to be crunchy. After half-hour of simmering, put off the pot from the heat, season to flavor, and blend till clean with a hand blender (aggregate for a splendidly silky soup).

4.  Decorate crème fraîche swirls and a sliver of blue cheese with glowing thyme leaves and pumpkin seeds.

5.  To taste, add salt and pepper.

6.  Serving idea: crusty bread

## Popcorn

Nothing tastes better at the same time as you want to lighten up at the couch and watch a movie than popcorn, whether or not candy or savory. This is a cute snack for you and the whole own family.

(4 Servings)

Ingredients

•1 Tablespoon 14.3g (0.Five ounces.) vegetable or sunflower oil

•50g or 1 ¾ Ounces of popping corn

To serve

•Honey

•Salt

•Butter

•Chocolate

•Powdered sugar

Method

1.     Add the oil and the kernels to a tremendous, heavy-bottomed pan with a respectable-fitting lid. (Using a pan with a heavy base will prevent the kernels from burning in the course of cooking.) Only upload ¼ of the advocated amount of corn kernels to the pan to permit for expansion.

2.   Cook the kernels of their skins until they start to "pop" and burst out of the pan at the

same time as maintaining the lid on and on occasion shaking it over medium warm temperature.

3. Take the pan off the variety, making sure that the popping has stopped, then switch the contents right right into a big bowl.

four. Sprinkle some powdered sugar, honey, or salt at the popcorn even as it's though heated.

five. You may additionally want to function a hint to the skillet as the butter melts and swirl it into the popcorn. Pour melted chocolate over the popcorn and permit it set for a unique treat.

Chocolate Fondue

Chocolate fondue is a fave of all. This simple dessert is the best justification for purchasing every body collectively for an fun, social nighttime. Fresh banana, pineapple, and strawberry chunks form delectable dunks for the decadent, creamy sauce. This rich chocolate fondue will wow your traffic, whether or not you are particular friends or hosting a quiet dinner for 2.

(4 Servings)

Ingredients

•three ¾ Cups or 110 g of sugar

•(a hundred and ten ml)(three.7 oz.) of Water

•14 Ounces (4 hundred g) chocolate (darkish, milk, or white)

To serve

•Grapes

•Pineapples

•Strawberries

•Marshmallows

•Bananas

Method

1.   In a medium-sized saucepan, warmness the water and sugar slowly until the sugar dissolves and a syrup paperwork.

2.   In a heatproof bowl, add the chocolate and harm it into quantities. Set the bowl over a pan of simmering water. (Avoid letting the bowl's base contact the water; doing so must motive the chocolate to seize and emerge as lumpy.)

three.   To create a clean sauce, combine the chocolate with the syrup and whisk with a timber spoon.

four.   Ensure that the sauce cools down a hint before serving because it is able to be noticeably pretty spiced. You can serve bite-sized quantities of glowing fruit or marshmallows with the aid of manner of dipping them in the sauce.

5.   A teaspoon of peppermint essence, some orange zest, the contents of a vanilla bean, or a tablespoon of Irish cream liqueur are some

extraordinary flavorings you can use in the sauce.

Spiced Banana Bread

Spiced banana bread with a pat of glowing butter is like manna from heaven and is a delectable cope with for breakfast, afternoon tea, or dessert. This moist banana bread might be an exceptional deal with over Christmas and Easter.

(12–15 slices regular with batch)

Ingredients

•55g of Unsalted butter, or 2 ounces..

•200g (7 oz) of Brown sugar

•1 Beaten egg

•three Mashed, overripe bananas, 82.Three ounces (250 g) self-elevating flour

•1 Salt shaker

• 2 Teaspoons (28.3g) (0.Nine oz.) of spices (a pinch of nutmeg and cinnamon)

• Grated 1 ¾ oz... (50 g) of dark chocolate

To serve (Optional)

• Butter

• Slices of banana

Method

1.   Set the oven's temperature to 350°F (a hundred 80°C, Gas four).

2.   A 7.Seventy five x 4 inch (19cm x 10cm) loaf pan ought to be greased or blanketed with parchment paper.

3.   Use a timber spoon or an electric whisk to mix the butter and sugar.

4.   Add the mashed bananas and the crushed egg to the aggregate.

## Chapter 7: The 5 Dimensions Of Hygge

Hygge is an mind-set. Sometimes I worry that we would forget that within the deluge of social media updates and brilliantly styled Instagram photos. It is a manner of being and taking within the global. Being more privy to the winning 2nd is a top notch approach to hook up with those feelings.

Each folks has a terrific technique for doing this, whether or not it consists of photos, meditation, cooking, drawing, or a few specific enjoyment or hobby pastime. There isn't always any want to exit and buy an high priced throw to begin gambling the hygge lifestyle; as an opportunity, sports activities sports that make us prevent and consider what we're doing and what is around us are a super manner to get began out!

The Taste Of Hygge

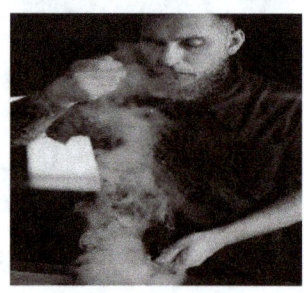

Because hygge frequently involves eating, the flavor is a crucial factor. And it can't be overly novel, unconventional, or complicated. Hygge almost usually has a familiar, sweet, and cushty flavor. Adding honey to tea makes it cozier and extra hyggelig. You can comply with icing to a cake to make it greater cushty. Additionally, you can upload wine on your stew to make it more hyggelig.

## The Sound Of Hygge

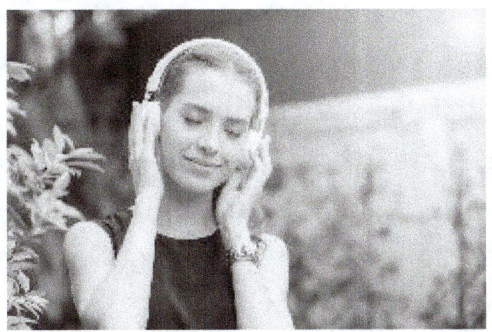

The maximum charming sounds are perhaps the tiny sparks and brief crackles of burning wood. But if you stay in an rental and can't have an open fireplace without walking a big chance of loss of existence, don't panic. Many noises have hyggelig features.

In truth, Hygge is specially characterized by manner of the shortage of noise, which permits you to pay interest even especially soft noises like rain at the roof, the wind blowing outside the window, the sound of wooden swaying inside the wind, or the creaks of wood planks that flex underneath your ft.

Hyggelig sounds also can embody someone cooking, knitting, or portray. Hygge's soundtrack will encompass any sound that inspires a steady feeling. For example, if you are interior and feel steady, the sound of thunder can be pretty hyggeligt; in case you are outdoor, now not a lot.

Smells Like Hygge

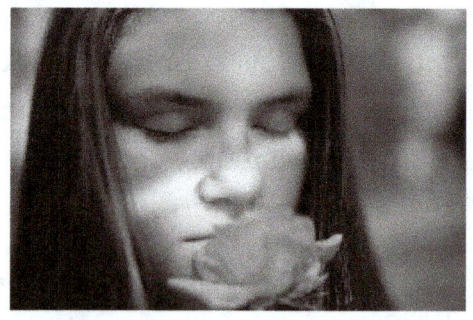

Have you ever professional a scent that transports you to a time frame or vicinity in that you felt consistent? Or professional a scent that, greater than a recollection, delivered again recollections of methods the world seemed to you as a toddler?

Another possibility is that effective smells elicit robust sentiments of protection and luxury, together with the scent of a bakery, the aroma of the apple wooden to your young adults outdoor, or perhaps the comforting aroma of your mother and father' home.

People's perceptions of what makes a scent hyggelig variety substantially because smells hyperlink modern situations to the ones that they have formerly related to that scent. The fragrance of cigarettes inside the morning can both make you experience unwell or offer you with a headache, counting on who you ask.

All of the hygge-inspired scents have one component in not unusual: they feature a reminder of protection and nurturing. We use odor to experience whether or not or no longer or now not some component is steady to eat, but we moreover use it to intuit whether or not a place is secure and the manner alert we have to be.

The fragrance of Hygge is the heady scent that tells you to region your shield down absolutely. The fragrance of cooking, the smell of a blanket you use at domestic, or the heady scent of an area we understand as steady can be very hyggeligt because it reminds us of a rustic of mind we expert while we felt absolutely secure.

What Does Hygge Feel Like?

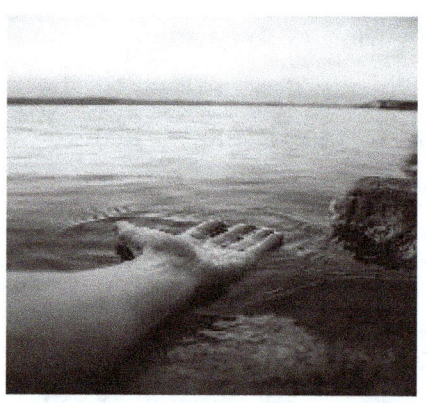

As I indicated, Hygge may be evoked thru letting your fingers waft over a wooden floor, spherical a warmth porcelain cup, or thru the hairs on a reindeer's skin. Old, exertions-sizeable hand made objects usually have a higher degree of coziness than newly produced gadgets.

And little subjects are usually cozier than huge ones. Denmark's motto is "The smaller, the extra hyggeligt," instead of the united states "The larger, the better." Nearly all the houses in Copenhagen are actually three or 4 reminiscences tall.

The hygge detail in those ancient systems is extra considerable than that during new homes composed of steel, glass, and concrete. Anything made via way of hand, together with gadgets product of wooden, ceramics, wool, leather-based, and unique materials, is considered hyggeligt. Although they may be if they're vintage sufficient, brilliant steel and glass aren't hyggeligt.

The hygge touch is interested by the herbal, rustic floor of things which might be flawed or have been or can be impacted thru manner of growing older. In addition, being warm temperature is not just like feeling warm temperature while indoors some issue heat in a chilly environment. It creates the effect that you are snug in a damaging putting.

Seeing Hygge

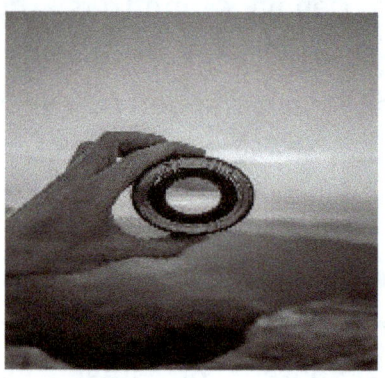

As we've already referred to, Hygge might be very lots about mild. Too masses brightness is not comfortable. Hygge, however, moreover emphasizes taking some time. You can take a look at this with the useful resource of watching languid motions, collectively with the lazily flickering flames of an open fireplace, lightly falling snow, or aqilokoq, due to the fact the Inuits might say.

In summary, hyggelige is defined as gradual, herbal movements and darkish, natural colors. It is not the sight of a smooth, properly-lit hospital or the presence of shifting site visitors. Slow, rustic, and dim is hygge.

## The Sixth Sense Of Hygge

The idea of Hygge is protection. Therefore, Hygge is a sign of self warranty for your surroundings and the human beings you're with. And the hygge sensation is an indication that you feel happy at the same time as someone advises you to comply with your gut intuition, which you have spread out your consolation region to consist of splendid human beings, and that you are feeling like you'll be absolutely actual with different human beings.

Hygge can be felt, heard, tasted, smelled, touched, and seen. However, Hygge is most importantly felt. Winnie-the-Pooh have become referenced at the beginning of the e-book, and I take into account his advice continues to be legitimate in recent times. You do no longer spell love. It's palpable. This brings us to the e-book's final problem, that is joy.

## Addicted To Hygge

While you should buy a cake, happiness can't, as a minimum in our brain's judgment, be offered. Open a espresso store's door on your thoughts. As quickly as you input, the welcoming fragrances from the whole thing at the counter tempt you, and on the identical time as you notice all of the pastries and desserts, you sense extremely joyful.

Your frame starts offevolved to experience euphoric as you are taking the primary piece of your chosen cake, that you have selected. Yes, that is a actual factor. But have you ever ever idea about why consuming sugary additives makes you so satisfied? There is a shape known as the nucleus accumbens within the basal forebrain.

It is a part of the thoughts's praise gadget and plays a massive element in reinforcement, motivation, and satisfaction. Like all vertebrates, we've got this tool because of the truth we have to enjoy sports activities activities like consuming and having intercourse. After all, they may be vital to the survival of our species.

A chemical is launched within the thoughts, and the signaling chemical dopamine is induced whilst you are engaged in an activity this is visible as pleasurable. Dopamine is launched in praise times from an area of the mind called the ventral tegmental vicinity, that's near the nucleus accumbens.

## Chapter 8: Everything You Need To Know About The History, Meaning, And Impacts Of Hygge

You have picked this e-book to examine because of the reality you need to reveal your life spherical, or improve the awesome of your life thru hygge. But earlier than delving into the whys and the hows, do you recognise what "hygge dwelling" exactly suggest? Are you acquainted about its foundational values and requirements?

Many people test hygge via without a doubt following the example of various people. They count on they need to do it as properly, sincerely in order that they emulate the practices of others without in truth expertise the cause at the back of the act. The trouble with this is the possibility of being disenchanted approximately the blessings of adopting hygge as a manner of existence. You would in all likelihood top notch be touching it on a superficial degree, consequently the outstanding outcomes that you may be looking ahead to have to most likely materialize on a lesser scale.

To clearly enjoy the hygge existence, learning its definitions, facts, and affects on societies and the sector in modern-day need to be the first step which you want to take.

Understanding the Definitions of Hygge Living

Hygge encompasses hundreds of factors so it couldn't be sufficiently defined in a unmarried phrase in the English language. A properly way to understand its that means is by way of manner of gaining knowledge of the middle values and concepts of hygge—comfort, companionship, rest, connection to nature, simplicity, and authenticity.

Comfort

Practicing hygge technique attempting to find comfort in various additives of your existence. When one achieves this, you'll be able to flow ahead at the same time as feeling happy and contented with the alternatives that you have made alongside the manner. Following this direction should then ultimately lead you to discovering the this means that of your lifestyles.

How is this possible?

In hygge, comfort is all approximately coziness. When you enjoy snug, the whole lot indoors you and round you feels right. For example:

o Feeling comfortable with your self approach that your interest is within the right here and now rather than the beyond or the future. You virtually like yourself, thereby allowing you to move with self assurance and a feel of purpose.

You specific positivity in the things you say and do. Through this, you are able remain degree-headed and comfortable, even if confronted with challenges on your lifestyles.

Nothing have to stop you from going after your desires and aspirations in existence. You are strongly related along with your thoughts, emotions, and spirituality, consequently providing you with an first-rate vicinity to begin about the course that you have to take.

o Spending time with fantastic humans is a crucial trouble of a hygge-based totally manner of lifestyles. As such, you want to discover ways to enjoy cushty with those spherical you. Doing so need to then allow you to construct close relationships which is probably useful to every person worried.

Being snug on the same time as inside the presence of different humans may be done even when you have a truely reserved person. Experts in hygge preserve in mind that this all starts with setting up proper eye touch with the character you're interacting with. This non-verbal gesture sends out a message which you are self-assured, no matter the manner you truly revel in internal.

At first, it can experience uncomfortable, but thru everyday exercising, you may be able to preserve eye touch with out lots effort from your detail. Just remember to keep away from staring an excessive amount of at one-of-a-kind humans due to the fact you will possibly purpose them to feel uncomfortable.

Inspiring comfort the diverse ones round you is considered as some other social detail of a hygge life-style. Your self-self guarantee attracts humans closer to you. Observing how you communicate and act has a bent to deliver out the first-rate in anybody round you. Ultimately, your effective outlook in life influences others to take at the same exercise.

o If you found you are secure and secured in your environment, then you may say that you are feeling comfortable to be in it. You can live there without fear of being harmed, and with out being agitated with the resource of the little subjects round you.

There are advantageous elements in existence in that you may no longer be able to feel genuinely snug in your surroundings right away. Moving to a modern-day home, journeying a distant places city, taking up a modern job—the ones situations require a fantastic time body to adjust and regain the feel of comfort you have got were given toward your environment.

Still, hygge calls with the intention to circulate beyond this adjustment length so you can constantly live this form of way of life. Later on, you'll examine in this ebook the manner to use the thoughts of hygge in an effort to enjoy snug, over again, collectively along side your environment.

Achieving consolation in the entirety you do can take lots of time and effort. However, as many practitioners of hygge must attest, this initiative is well worth given its numerous advantages for you and the people you care about.

Companionship

Hygge is all approximately supporting each other at the route closer to happiness. Making a addiction out of being useful in choice to being self-focused want to bring about a greater substantial existence, and additional snug critiques for each person.

No you probably can undergo life all on their non-public. Throughout your lifetime, you'll connect to specific human beings to various tiers. Some could likely come to be being your close to pals and mentors, while others should come into your existence as soon as however in no way to be seen yet again. Many people are going to engage with you, no matter their ordinary impact on you. Therefore, attempt to make the maximum out of your moment together with them.

Feeling the warm temperature of companionship with the people costly to you and with the individuals who would in all likelihood come and skip on your existence gives you greater than just cushty opinions. It is also going to the touch you on a non secular degree. The things you can research from them should assist you to increase in processes that you could no longer be able to acquire this in your very non-public.

For example, random acts of kindness, particularly the ones via manner of accomplished through strangers, is a superb supply of such instructions. By witnessing or experiencing this for yourself, you may be able to take a look at the cost of paying it forward. Being type to someone proper now—with out a need a few thing in move lower back proper away—ought to provide you with a risk to experience the joy of receiving help from sudden property. However, the actual essence of companionship, in phrases of hygge, pertains to the act of extending assist to others out of your private will—without or with reaping blessings you.

Hygge does not moreover good deal the truth that there are positive troubles in lifestyles which you might probably ought to face by myself that allows you to investigate and develop from them. Resolving your non-public issues without counting on others is a commendable act. Asking for assist from others, however, does not lessen its importance. Life can difficult as it is, so why make it more difficult thru way of ignoring or refusing the assist that extraordinary humans have to offer you with?

Companionship in hygge approach loving and being concerned for others unconditionally. It does not ask or want, however it gives willingly and wholeheartedly. Through this, you could create a sturdy feel of togetherness that promotes increase and development indoors all of us worried.

 Relaxation

Nowadays, nearly each person unearths themselves dashing thru the day without ever taking a pause to realize their reviews and the things round them. If you usually have some thing to worry about, or a few factor that desires to be completed at the soonest time viable, then you simply are probable this kind of humans.

Hygge, but, promotes mindfulness and the proper fee of time. Yes, you want to hold in mind the critical topics to your life, but that does not endorse which you want to continuously strain your self to finish the whole lot in file time.

Find the time to take it sluggish, even at least some instances a day. You can do so through using making it a factor to revel in your first cup of espresso for the day. Staying a hint longer within the bath earlier than going to bed also may be a incredible exercising of hygge. Take it sluggish in playing those clean subjects due to the reality you can end up regretting no longer doing so afterward.

Connection to Nature

Though hygge is generally associated with topics that you could do inside your home, it moreover touches at the attractions, sounds, aromas, and experiences that you can revel in from nature. You can be capable of appreciate the ones via way of way of easy, fun engagements along with going out for a stroll in the park, reading your favored e-book underneath the color of a tree, or preserving yourself hydrated at the seashore with the useful resource of eating coconut juice right now from the shell.

You also can hook up with nature through getting your blood pumping thru thrilling sports activities, like playing football out within the sun, snowboarding within the mountains, or swimming in the sea.

Winter would possibly possibly dispose of most of the greeneries, but that does not mean which you could not get to practice hygge. Keeping and tending to 3 potted vegetation in your property may want to permit you to understand the easy delights that nature has to provide.

Simplicity

Hygge covers the easy topics in existence. Studies show that the Danes have a tendency to area a lesser value on materials and luxuries in comparison to others. What they treasure greater are their private research and their relationships with own family individuals and buddies.

This form of thinking permits them to stay a smooth existence that expenses masses inexpensive than hoarding topics or preserving up with converting tendencies in fashion, generation, among others. For example, going out on a hike at the side of your near pals can be an outstanding opportunity to create lasting memories that would moreover promote a better appreciation and reference to the surroundings.

Quiet moments like enjoyable thru the fireplace with cup of warm chocolate also are considered as hygge due to the fact easy self-care measures are truly as critical as traumatic for others.

Authenticity

In hygge, putting a first-rate price on comfort, rest, and simplicity does now not mean that you have to take shortcuts whenever you pass. Rather, you need to aim for authenticity in the whole lot you do.

Take for instance the trouble of indulging yourself together with your preferred comfort meals. Eating it'd convey you pleasure, but you could get plenty extra from the revel in via seeking to create it from scratch.

Fortunately, most of the famous comfort ingredients are pretty easy to put together, because of this making it less complicated that lets in you to discover ways to attain this. To get you started out out on this, chapter ____ of this ebook gives severa exceptional hygge recipes which you have to actually try making yourself.

You can also moreover take this to the following diploma by way of getting your self onboard with the farm-to-table fashion. Skip the grocery store, and head as a substitute to the local farmers' market. Better but, attempt planting and tending to three herbs and small vegetation in your property so you can harvest your very private elements.

Hygge technique selecting authenticity over consolation, on every occasion relevant. Aside from the delight of laboring over some thing that subjects to you, doing so may need to allow to take higher care of your frame in the long run.

All in all, hygge is ready enhancing one's exceptional of lifestyles with the useful resource of organising and keep a very good relationship with the self, with different human beings, and with the surroundings.

Considering the ones definitions of hygge, it need to now not wonder you that its practitioners, especially the Danes, are seemed because the happiest human beings within the global. But how did hygge come into existence within the first region? Where did all of it begin, and the manner did it turn out to be one of the maximum famous manner of life traits for the duration of the globe?

To answer the ones questions and extra, here's a quick examine of the history of hygge and its affects on modern society and worldwide in standard.

Discovering the History of Hygge

The pronunciation of hygge is not the best confounding issue of the phrase. Experts have attempted to trace its roots, however up until now, no consensus has been reached aside from the truth that the concept regarded first someday within the nineteenth century. Here are a number of the common speculations about the origins of hygge:

o "hyggja"

•Source Language: Old Norse

•Meaning: "to suppose"

o "hugr" or "hug"

•Source Language: Old Norse

•Meaning: "mind", "interest", "temper" or "soul"

o "hugge"

•Source Language: Unknown, however most in all likelihood Old Norse

•Meaning: "to embrace"

o "hygga"

•Source Language: Old Norse

•Meaning: "to comfort"

o "hycgan"

•Source Language: Old English

•Meaning: "to endure in thoughts" or "to suppose"

These terms seemed in 19th century Danish literature, however they had been culturally applicable inside the Scandinavian international locations. At the time, Denmark were reeling from its loss inside the Second Prussian War that took away the duchies of Holstein and Schleswig from them. As a cease cease result, the Danes began out suffering from a large financial decline.

In response to this monetary downturn, the country rallied behind the idea of regaining what has been lost with the useful resource of rebuilding from inside. Their popularity shifted to growing their groups and fostering their relationships with one another as opposed to interacting with other worldwide locations.

The strategy has set up to be pretty effective as it grade by grade increased Denmark, alongside facet its Scandinavian pals, because the happiest and wealthiest global places inside the global. As such, the exercising of hygge piques the interest of various societies which might be experiencing large shifts of their subculture, politics, and economies.

Appreciating the Various Impacts of Hygge Across Different Societies in the World

The concept of hygge has been in life since the early 1800's, however it changed into first-rate in mid-2010's that the relaxation of the area stuck wind of it. This upward push in popularity maintains to surge for the duration of unique structures—blogs, social media, magazines, and books—for this reason allowing hygge to head beyond the regulations imposed via language and geography.

Case in factor, the time period itself have become included in some "Word of Year" lists in 2016. This uptrend in its utilization most probable stems from the dozens of books and articles which have been published specially in the US and the United Kingdom. Several manner of lifestyles experts raved approximately it that, in 2017, Pinterest diagnosed hygge as one of the most up to date décor developments among its clients. Up to at the triumphing time, humans in Twitter and Instagram hold to post hygge-associated photographs, and to talk about what makes a few factor hygge.

Proponents of a way of lifestyles primarily based on hygge did not discover this phenomenon surprising, for the reason that its center characteristics revolve around the pursuit of comfort and happiness. Its get right of entry to into the mainstream interest of severa international places mirror the shift of interest towards what's happening internal their international places in region of what is going on out of doors their borders.

This fashion can be positioned gambling out in a high scale within the US and the United Kingdom. The Republican advertising advertising campaign at some point of america presidential election of 2016 focused throughout the idea of creating their u.S. Of america "first-rate again" by using using prioritizing nationalistic pursuits in choice to putting in and maintaining international partnerships. Meanwhile, in the UK, majority of the citizens have voted on a referendum that would separate UK from the European Union.

Given those primary political upheavals, how does hygge have an effect on the way of existence of the human beings dwelling inside the course of these uncertain instances?

At the maximum number one level, hygge promotes happiness and togetherness. Pursuing the ones values permit individuals to benefit the energy and energy of will to triumph over the worrying conditions that come their way. Furthermore, they might in a function be able to offer assist and encouragement to the ones round them, for this reason developing a sense of belongingness that could stand the blows of the unexpected adjustments in life that lie beyond one's control.

The influences of hygge furthermore extends past the self, domestic, and community. It also can appreciably modify the way humans paintings for a living. Though it could sound counterintuitive for societies that promote lively competition, practising hygge at paintings approach aiming for maximum exceptional art work-existence stability. Rather fear approximately promotions and paychecks, the point of interest need to be on constructing well strolling relationships with every other, and enhancing the running surroundings into turning into a chilled and conducive area for questioning and creativity.

As the arena maintains to talk about on whether or no longer nationalism or globalism is the future, the idea of hygge persists and widens its scope of have an impact on amongst folks who are searching out for happiness and luxury in their very very own little methods.

Having found the definitions, statistics, and influences of hygge, you might be thinking that the concept isn't always surely unique. After all, it's far herbal for humans to look for solace and happiness of their life. Your very non-public manner of existence may furthermore have its version of a hygge-like lifestyle. Here are a few examples of the well-known thoughts that undergo brilliant similarities with the which means, origins, or packages of hygge.

 Fika

Pronunciation: FEE-kah

Many take into account this as one of the middle practices of the Swedes. Essentially, this is Swedish model of a coffee smash. It entails enjoyable refreshments and high-quality snacks, mixed with feelings of contentment.

Fika is basically based absolutely on the belief on artwork and spoil instances in Sweden. The human beings there do not forget that one have to no longer paintings more than what is required. Taking a wreck at distinctive factors of the day is not taken into consideration a waste of time. Rather, it's far considered as a manner of preserving a healthy balance in a single's existence.

Through this, you'll be capable of moderate your existence nicely. You is probably able to exercising self-care and connect with your own family and buddies, on the equal time as making sure a excellent regular universal performance at art work.

To workout fika, set apart some time each day to hang around with the people you want and care approximately. Look for a quiet and interesting place wherein you may entice up with them over espresso and pastries.

As you can inform via now, fika and hygge promotes the idea of slowing down and appreciating the splendid vibes added approximately through the presence of various human beings. Both necessities need you to live inside the moment, and revel in the easy subjects in lifestyles.

Friluftsliv

Pronunciation: unfastened-LOOFTS-leev

This Norwegian time period, which genuinely method "loose air lifestyles", relates to the act of connecting with nature with the useful resource of taking part in numerous outside activities, collectively with skiing, sledding, trekking or perhaps virtually strolling or jogging across the park. Norway, despite the entirety, is domestic to numerous nature spots that hundreds and thousands of locals and tourists visit every year.

However, frilutsliv is not pretty a whole lot spending time outside. It is a manner of residing, just like hygge. This concept encourages humans to practice mindfulness to be one with nature. Ultimately, frilutsliv may additionally need to will can help you achieve a higher degree of hobby, and to installation a stronger connection with your spirituality.

How do Norwegians exercise this kind of life-style?

First, they make it a issue to educate the idea to youngsters. Beyond the house and the college, children are regularly given the threat to apply frilutsliv in order that they may hold to do in the course of their lifetime.

You do no longer need to live or live in Norway definitely to carry out that as properly. You can also workout frilutsliv everywhere you're, so long as you learn how to properly admire the time you spend out in nature. This does now not suggest which you need to schedule a hike in the mountains, or go snowboarding every weekend. Simple acts, collectively with taking a deep breath of easy air at the identical time as you're out on a walk, can also permit you to revel in in contact with the area spherical you.

Friluftliv does now not advocate that you want to do the entirety by myself so you can better connect to nature. You also can consist of it at the side of your circle of relatives and buddies. Feel unfastened to participate in group outside sports—just make sure to have in thoughts of the topics which you are doing with your companions.

When you spend time at the beach, set aside a bit of time to revel in the warmth of the solar in your pores and skin, breathe within the sea breeze, and experience the sand beneath your ft. Doing so may relax your body, calm your thoughts, and raise your spirits.

 Gemütlichkeit

Pronunciation: guh-MYOOT-lik-kayt

Much like hygge, the German concept of gemutlichkeit refers to feeling warm temperature and luxury while inside the agency corporation of different human beings. It can be practiced inside the home, at the same time as at artwork, or throughout social sports. However, in contrast to 365 days-round hygge residing, this essentially applies all through the iciness months best.

Experts be given as actual with that the difficult cold outside had driven the Germans to create a warm temperature and cushty surroundings anywhere they may be staying. For instance, setting out with the people you have had been given dined with is considered as gemutlichkeit, so long as anyone is having a grand time. So does playing a classical piano piece while your family listen and drink tea. In this experience, you could say that gemutlichkeit is all about spending first-rate time in a comfortable environment with the people you care approximately.

Introverts may additionally moreover additionally enjoy practicing this concept thru the usage of doing all your preferred pursuits. Reading your preferred e-book through way of the hearth, or immersing yourself with 1000-piece puzzle and a pitcher of wine may additionally need to produce the right surroundings that gemutlichkeit is promoting.

## Chapter 9: Understanding Why You Should Pursue Happiness Like A Danish

Numerous research executed about the amount of happiness exhibited via the Danish humans have validated that they owe a whole lot of it from their workout of hygge. The attribution of pride, warmth, and comfort to this shape of manner of existence have lead many human beings to agree with that it would furthermore flip their life round.

But how precisely so?

Though arguably the most well-known gain of a hyggelig manner of life is getting to experience the clean pleasures in lifestyles collectively along with your family, there are masses of other advantages that you can expect from taking the initiative to use its necessities to various additives of your each day living.

To higher apprehend and admire the consequences of hygge on a personal degree, right proper right here are the pinnacle physical, intellectual, and emotional benefits of adopting this form of way of lifestyles:

For the Body

Hygge promotes emotions of safety and calm. When sustained for an less expensive time period, this shape of surroundings enables the body to modify therefore. Rather than being always prepared for moments of stress and danger, the frame might be able to lighten up and refocus its assets on it others talents, together with healing, self-cleansing, and fighting off bacteria and viruses.

Upon accomplishing this physical kingdom, you will be able to acquire the subsequent bodily advantages of hygge:

o Lower Levels of Stress Hormone

The human frame is hardwired to react accordingly to numerous forms of threat. Back in ancient times, this mechanism enabled the survival of mankind in competition to predators and harmful forces of danger. Such threats did no longer actually disappear over the years, however as a substitute they developed in strategies that drastically have an effect on one's regular residing.

For example, absolutely everyone goes thru the trouble of meeting the dreams from one-of-a-kind factors of life—searching after the family, tackling a heavy workload, or looming due dates for bills. Though those stressors are pretty one in all a type from warding off wild beasts, the body acknowledges those as threats to at least one's life.

When this takes place, the body releases cortisol, the principle strain hormone, and adrenaline into the blood flow into. This may additionally then stop end result to:

•Elevated heart fee

•Increased blood stress

•Higher degree of glucose within the blood

•Altered immune system

•Suppressed digestive tool, reproductive system, and cell increase

These changes within the frame allow a person to have greater strength for movement and thoughts characteristic. More physical sources are also allotted for the repair of cells and tissues. Ultimately, the stress hormones sell skills that would aid in a combat-or flight state of affairs, and repress those that do not make a contribution tons or in any respect.

Once the stressor has been removed or minimized, the outcomes of cortisol and adrenaline moreover deplete till the frame has been restored to its normal functioning. However, many people do no longer get to de-pressure themselves prolonged sufficient for the cool all the way right down to show up.

Extended exposure to strain hormones have a propensity to be significantly disruptive inside the direction of simply each essential physical feature. As such, it might located surely each person at excessive danger of growing:

- Various cardiovascular ailments

- Weight gain

- Mental impairments

- Digestive problems

- Inability to sleep

- Depression

- Anxiety

- Severe headaches

Given the ones in all likelihood effects of overexposure to pressure hormones, it's miles essential to learn how to address stressors in a healthy way.

The exercise of hygge is considered as one of the more powerful techniques of doing so. At its center, this type of way of existence promotes the idea of getting rid of 1's self from situations that might be emotionally overwhelming, and instead, focusing on the matters that would make one happy.

These thoughts are pretty clean to apply than you may probably anticipate. Compared to specific life-style tendencies, hygge does not require a good buy try or money. In fact, the lots less you spend, the greater hyggelig your existence is probably. Examples of hyggelig moments that would drastically lessen the quantity of pressure hormones include but are not confined to:

•Sitting beside a hearth

•Baking cookies, desserts, and certainly one of a type kinds of pastries

•Having an intimate dinner with circle of relatives and buddies

•Snuggling below a thick blanket with the one you love

•Wearing a comfortable cardigan

•Going on a nature hike

Essentially, hygge is all approximately being type to your self, to the people round you, and to the surroundings. Appreciating the clean pleasures in existence is a exceptional way of giving your body enough time to get higher from the results of strain hormones.

o Better Quality of Sleep

Sleep performs an crucial function in attaining proper bodily, intellectual, and emotional well being. During this period, the body have to rest and repair itself. Growth and development additionally gets a lift, specifically among kids.

The right amount of sleep varies constant with age agency, but on a mean, a seven-hour sleep may also moreover need to do wonders for the frame. Failing to acquire the prescribed amount have to lead to sleep deprivation, which in turn affects the following:

•Vulnerability towards illnesses, together with coronary heart disease, stroke, excessive blood pressure, and diabetes

•Memory and focus

•Control over temper and feelings

•Performance on the same time as conscious

•Personal safety

Getting the quantity right is crucial, however insufficient if you have attained it thru synthetic manner, like taking sleeping capsules, or if you woke feeling tired after a compelled sleep. The extremely good of your sleep subjects virtually as lots due to the fact the type of hours you've got slept.

Health experts propose precise techniques to gain enough correct-splendid sleep. For instance:

•Establishing and following a ritual in advance than going to bed

•Keeping the equal sleep time desk every day, regardless if it's miles a weekday or the weekends

•Refraining from the use of any virtual tool at the least one hour earlier than bedtime

These techniques have demonstrated to be powerful for masses humans. Hygge, however, boosts the expected final results from taking on all or any of these tasks. It also can make it less complex so one can create an extended-lasting addiction out of those sleep-inducing behaviors.

Applying hygge to the manner you sleep is quite easy to do. For many, it starts offevolved offevolved with the aid of manner of turning the mattress room into a chilled sleep sanctuary. Anything that would make both your frame and mind enjoy at rest may be placed somewhere in this location—fluffy pillows, knitted blankets, or scented candles. Having the ones items in the bed room ought to help motive the ordinary release of serotonin, the primary hormone that is related to a restful night time time.

Once the excellent setting has been performed, hyggelig practices may additionally need to shape a part of your regular drowsing ritual to in addition loosen up the frame and the thoughts. Here are some of the as an alternative advocated activities that you ought to really don't forget:

•Taking a nice, long warmth bathtub

•Listening to fun song

•Performing meditation or mindfulness physical video games

•Writing down the things you are grateful for in a every day magazine

Take check, however, that hygge does not provide an entire assure that it'd remedy the napping issues which you have, such as insomnia or sleep paralysis. At great, it is able to assist you create an environment that could boom your opportunities of having the best length and fine of sleep for you. For greater intense and continual sleep-related problems, you need to are trying to find the recommendation of a clinical expert.

o Improved Weight Management

Hygge isn't a healthy dietweight-reduction plan neither is it a weight loss degree. What it does for weight management is beautify the way you eat, sleep workout, and entertain your self. It might in all likelihood now not make you shed ten kilos right off the bat, but operating in the direction of hygge will assist you hold your frame in properly shape. For instance:

– Being aware of what you consume and drink

Taking the time to get pride from and apprehend each chew and sip will assist you adjust your eating behavior. Rather than making do with frozen meals and speedy meals devices—both of which incorporate excessive stages of sodium and trans-fat—you may be more aware about the belongings you consume each day.

Furthermore, chewing the food slowly would increase your ingesting time. According to experts, doing so might probable make you revel in complete even if you have not but eaten a vast quantity of food.

–Turning the act of eating proper into a completely particular occasion

Due to the severa desires of present day life, a few people might be tempted to consume a brief meal within the the front of the TV instead of cooking and sharing food with the people you care approximately.